At Face Value

At Face Value

My Struggle with a Disfiguring Cancer

Terry Healey

Grateful acknowledgment is made to the following for their permission to reprint excerpts from songwriter and singer Corey Hart's song "Never Surrender": Excerpt from "Never Surrender", written by Corey Hart 1985. ©Published by Liesse Publishing/ Harco Productions. Used by permission.

The names of many people mentioned in this book have been changed. All of the medical doctor's names mentioned in this book have been changed. Names of any doctor's included in this book are intended to be fictional names, and any similarities in name are purely coincidental.

This book was printed in the United States of America.

To order additional copies of this book, contact:
Xlibris Corporation
1-888-7-XLIBRIS
www.Xlibris.com
Orders@Xlibris.com

Contents

Acknowledgments 7

PROLOGUE 9

CHAPTER ONE
Dead End on Easy Street 11

CHAPTER TWO
Back to School 19

CHAPTER THREE
College With My Eyes Closed 29

CHAPTER FOUR
Positive Thinking 35

CHAPTER FIVE
Brutal Reality 41

CHAPTER SIX
The Waiting Game 50

CHAPTER SEVEN
The Tumor Board 61

CHAPTER EIGHT
Anticipation 72

CHAPTER NINE
Making Me 'Streetable' 83

CHAPTER TEN
Encounters with the Outside World 113

CHAPTER ELEVEN
The Re-entry Program 147

CHAPTER TWELVE
Trying To Fit In Again 170

CHAPTER THIRTEEN
Starts and Stops 199

CHAPTER FOURTEEN
Reconstruction . . . Finally 219

CHAPTER FIFTEEN
New Challenges 241

CHAPTER SIXTEEN
A Better Life 255

Acknowledgments

I am grateful to many, many people, without whose support this book would never have been completed.

For inspiration to write this book: Susan Wittig Albert, whose uncanny ability to believe I had a story that needed to be told, even though she didn't know me. Rob Healey, my brother, who never stopped believing in my book and me. Sue Healey, my wife, who supported me despite the endless hours this book took away from our time together. Peter Jackson, who encouraged me that my story had to be told. Diane Inman, the best English teacher I ever had, who encouraged writing from the heart.

For encouragement during my treatment and unending love and support during my reconstruction and thereafter: Patricia Healey, my mother; Donald Healey, my father; Steve Healey, Brian Healey and Rob Healey, my three brothers; Tyler Higgins, Dave Lunceford and Tom Witter, my dearest friends.

For editorial assistance: Monica Faulkner and Bridget Moar.

For cover design: Laura Chambliss, the most talented designer and artist I know.

For legal advice: Andrew Gold.

For helping me to stay alive to write this: All the wonderful doctors and nurses at UCSF.

PROLOGUE

It was a beautiful Saturday in September 1985, and my fraternity was preparing for a big party we'd be hosting that evening. Late that afternoon, and after numerous cold beers, a group of us wandered out to the courtyard from the inside bar to get some fresh air. Pretty soon, we were all heckling one another and started giving each other short jabs to the shoulders and chest – all in fun. I went for the takedown and knocked my buddy Chip down onto the concrete, where we began wrestling and rolling around.

All of a sudden, blood started trickling out of my nose. I wasn't overly surprised because I'd always gotten frequent nosebleeds.

"Oh, dude, I'm sorry," Chip said, helping me up. "I didn't mean to hit your nose."

"Don't worry. It's no big deal," I said.

But suddenly I wasn't interested in horsing around anymore. The bleeding was getting heavier, and what scared me was that I didn't remember him hitting me in the nose at all.

I covered my nose and mouth with my hands and ran up to my room. I dashed to the sink, turned on the cold water, and splashed water over my face.

The bleeding stopped almost immediately, but when I looked in the mirror, I felt my stomach cramp in panic. I could see an ivory-colored lump sticking up from the lower section of my right nostril. It seemed as if the bleeding was coming from that area. This didn't seem like my run-of-the-mill nosebleed.

A year earlier, the doctors had told me that they had gotten rid of all of the cancer. But now, I started wondering. Had it come back?

CHAPTER ONE

Dead End on Easy Street

It had all begun a year earlier, in Berkeley, California, on a sunny but chilly Saturday morning in October 1984. I was twenty and a junior majoring in political science at the University of California at Berkeley, commonly known as "Cal". I was president of the Zeta Psi fraternity, also known as the Zete House, a fraternity more famous for its parties than for its members' academic achievements.

My mother, father, and three brothers were all on hand for the big game between the California Golden Bears and the University of Southern California Trojans at Memorial Stadium. My mother was treasurer of the Zete mothers' club, which was putting on a fundraising luncheon as the mothers did every year. It would be a joyful day with plenty of food and drink.

It would also be the day that an offhand remark by my oldest brother Steve would change my life forever.

*   *   *

I got up at about ten, in plenty of time for the start of the festivities at eleven, when we would start serving beer, wine, and gin fizzes to Zete alumni, friends, parents—and ourselves. As president, I was obligated to be on the scene to greet everyone.

My brother Steve, who had also been a Zete at Cal several years earlier, knocked on my door just before eleven. While I was getting dressed, we brought each other up to date on what we had been up to. An album by the Cal marching band was playing on my stereo.

I gave myself a final look in the mirror, then turned to face him. "I'm ready to go."

Steve squinted at me. "Hey, Terry, what's going on with your nose?"

"What?"

"Take a look. Your right nostril looks like it's flared out."

"What are you talking about?" I went back to the mirror and took a look. He was right. I had never noticed it, but my right nostril did look bigger than the left one. "Well, it's probably nothing," I shrugged. "Let's go grab a gin fizz."

*   *   *

I was twenty. No twenty-year-old ever thinks seriously about being sick, and I was no different. At least, not then.

John was one of my closest Zete House friends and drinking buddies, and he never hesitated to make personal comments. After dinner a week or so after the Cal-USC game, he and I went to his room to play some music and talk for a while before heading off to the library. John had an ability to focus on many things at once. He could play his electric guitar along with whatever song was playing and carry on a conversation at the same time.

"Hey, Heals," he said. "I don't mean to be rude, but I've been noticing something odd about your nose. Is everything okay?"

Not again, I thought. "Yeah," I replied, feeling a bit defensive. "Everything's fine. It's just a pimple or something."

I told him I was going to go study at the library, and we agreed to meet up at 'Manny's', a local bar, later. I had shrugged off his question, but as soon as he left and I went up to my room to get my backpack, I also took another look in the mirror.

I felt around the area and discovered a small, hard mass behind my right upper lip. What was going on? Maybe I ought to have my dentist look at it.

But it took two more seemingly minor incidents before I finally decided to act.

The first was when I picked up my new student identification card in Sproul Hall, the administration building. I glanced at the card, then stood still and took a closer look. The distortion on the right side of my nose was so obvious that I couldn't believe I hadn't been aware of it before.

I touched my nose and cheek and felt the small mass again. But it didn't hurt or feel strange in any way, so it couldn't be anything serious. Whatever it was would go away before long. I was sure of it.

The second incident occurred a few days later when my friend Sally stopped by with some pictures from a party she had taken me to a few weeks earlier.

I studied the photos. "Did you notice how lopsided my nose looks?" I asked her. As I waited for her response, I could feel my heart begin to beat faster and faster.

"What do you mean?" She looked puzzled.

I shoved one of the photos at her. "Look."

She glanced at it. "Oh, that's nothing," she said. But somehow I couldn't believe that she hadn't noticed anything.

We spent a few more minutes rehashing the party, but as soon as she left I went back to the mirror and felt around again. The lump was still there. A cyst, or a tumor? I wondered.

I tried to reassure myself by reminding myself that my mother had had a couple of tumors, one in her neck and one on her ovary. Both had been removed, and both had been benign. Everything always turned out okay.

But I decided to get whatever it was looked at. By now, three weeks had passed and the lump was still there. It made sense for me to go to my regular dentist because it felt as if most of the lump was above my upper front teeth and in my palate. So I made an appointment for the following week.

*   *   *

My dentist gave me a good looking-over and x-rayed the area.

"I think you should see an ear, nose, and throat specialist," he told me. "I don't think it's serious. Probably just a cyst."

A few days later, I drove to Oakland for my first appointment with the specialist, Dr. Tom Kernan. He was a balding, middle-aged man with an affable manner.

"I think you're overreacting," he told me with a smile after a brief examination. "It's probably nothing more than a pimple. I suggest that you apply hot compresses to the side of your nose three times a day for a few days until it rises to the surface. I'll also prescribe you a decongestant."

I felt humiliated, as if he thought I was being a hypochondriac. "I've had pimples before," I said, "and I really don't think that's what this is."

"I still think it's a pimple. Use the compresses. Come back in three weeks if there's no change, but in the meantime, try not to worry."

Three weeks later, the lump was still there.

This time my visit to the doctor's office took a more serious tone. "I'm pretty sure it's a cyst, or a benign tumor," Kernan told me. "I want to keep an eye on it for another month or so before we start talking about doing a biopsy on it."

*   *   *

Later on, people asked me why Kernan waited so long, and why I didn't go to another doctor. I don't know why he waited. Maybe he was reluctant to act too quickly when he wasn't sure what he was dealing with, especially if surgery would be involved. Why run the risk of scarring someone's face if in his professional experience most such conditions went away by themselves?

And it didn't occur to me to look for another doctor because I was too young to have had much experience with doctors or medical treatment. My dentist had referred me to Kernan, suggesting he was very qualified to examine and treat me. It wasn't until later that I would begin to realize that doctors are people too, and that they don't always have all the answers.

*   *   *

When the lump was still there a month after my second office visit, Kernan recommended a biopsy. He scheduled it at Providence Hospital in Oakland in mid-December, over my Christmas break. The timing was good, because it was the start of Christmas break, and my six-month term as fraternity president was completed with the end of the fall semester.

I felt completely calm and fearless that day. It never occurred to me that the "thing," whatever it was, might be malignant. The procedure took forty-five minutes, and all I needed was a local anesthetic. I didn't talk with Kernan afterwards because he left right away, apparently for another surgery.

The pathologist told me that it would take a couple of days to get the results from the tumor biopsy. But when he referred to it as a "tumor", his choice of words clarified to me immediately that we definitely weren't talking about a cyst.

Then, a few days later, Kernan called and told me that it would take a bit longer to get the results. It didn't occur to me to question the delay, but again, I was too young to be too concerned.

*   *   *

It was almost the end of January, five weeks after the biopsy, before Kernan phoned me in my room at the fraternity.

"I'd like you to come in and see me," he said.

This was a bad sign. My heart started racing, and I felt sick to my stomach. If my case was closed, why was he asking me to come in?

"When?" I asked.

"The sooner the better," he said.

"This afternoon?"

"Yes, that'd be fine. How about 4:00?"

"Okay." I hung up and took several deep breaths. I was still hoping for a positive outcome, but I knew I now had to prepare myself for bad news. I could be strong, I reassured myself.

*   *   *

I left my afternoon class early to make the appointment. After I checked in with Dr. Kernan's receptionist, a nurse immediately led me into an examining room. I perched myself on the waxy white paper covering the examining table. A few moments later, Dr. Kernan came in followed by an assistant who I learned later was working on a fellowship under him.

"Hi, Terry." Dr. Kernan shook my hand, then took a step back as if he had forgotten something. He kept backing up until I thought he was going to leave the room, but finally he stopped. He was gazing at the floor, and I realized that he was too nervous to look me in the eye.

"Well, uh . . . Terry . . . uh . . ."

I knew what he was going to say, even though he was having trouble getting the words out.

The assistant spoke up. "What the doctor's trying to tell you is . . ." He sounded rather like a son who knows what his aged father is trying to say but also knows that the father can no longer get the words out. " . . . Your tumor's malignant. It's a fibrosarcoma. But since we caught it in the early stages, it's unlikely that you'll have to worry about a recurrence."

Although I had spent the hours since Kernan's call preparing myself for this news, the truth was still cruel. But I wasn't going to let myself speculate. Not just yet.

"I understand," I said after a moment. "What's the next step?"

As I spoke, I realized that I was more embarrassed about Kernan's inability to tell me the news than I was upset to learn that I had cancer.

"I'm really sorry to have to tell you this," Kernan said, "but we feel positive that we can catch this thing."

I felt relieved that he was finally able to speak to me directly, although it was obviously still a struggle for him. He didn't seem like he had much experience delivering bad news.

"So you're going to have to go back in and get the rest of it?" I asked. "You didn't remove all of it the last time?"

"Yes. We need to make sure that all the fibers are removed. When we did the biopsy, we removed all that we could see of the tumor, but because it's malignant, we have to be sure that the margins are clean. One of the reasons it took so long to diagnose your tumor was that fibrosarcomas don't normally occur in the head and neck area. They typically grow in the bone and muscle in the legs."

Suddenly I could feel the news sinking in.

I had a malignant tumor.

A malignant tumor was serious. And not only was it malignant, it was a rare type of malignancy. I didn't know it then, but I had just taken the first step of a journey that would turn out to be the biggest challenge of my life so far. This journey would take me down many paths, and I would later realize that it would never truly end. For when someone is diagnosed with cancer, it's a life changing as well as a life-threatening event, and nothing is ever exactly the same again.

＊　　＊　　＊

That day, however, I had no idea what was in store. My attitude was, okay, I had cancer, but I wasn't about to waste time moping about it. I was going to fight it and beat it, and I couldn't wait to start.

"All right, then, let's set up the next surgery," I said.

CHAPTER TWO

Back to School

When I left Kernan's office, it was almost dinner time. I had told a couple of my friends about the appointment, and, knowing that they would ask me how it had gone, I decided to skip dinner at the fraternity and go for a drive through the Berkeley hills.

As I drove, I contemplated my future. Maybe I would have to drop out of school. Maybe I was going to die. I cried softly as I drove the winding roads above the Berkeley campus. As the winter twilight deepened into darkness, I drove back to the campus and parked near LaVal's Pizza Northside, away from the more undergraduate frequented Southside La Val's.

I ordered a pizza and a beer and took my time eating. I knew that I was basically burning up as much time as I could so that I wouldn't have to face anyone or answer any questions. I didn't feel guilty about not calling my parents or my brothers because I hadn't told them about the appointment that day to begin with. Finally, I decided to go back to the Zete house. If anyone asked, I would say that everything was fine. Fortunately, I didn't run into anyone who knew I'd been at the doctor. I called it an early night, but I tossed and turned all night and got very little sleep.

*   *   *

The next morning, I got up early and walked over to the Newman Center. I was raised a Roman Catholic, and prayer had always been a part of my life. Although I was confident that I could handle this challenge, I also felt I needed help from God.

That morning, I prayed for the strength I would need to beat my cancer. I prayed that I would sustain my will to live. I prayed that my family would stay strong and that my parents would be able to handle the emotional and financial stress that my disease might cause them. I prayed for my brothers' support and for the support of my friends.

When I left the church, I stopped and dipped my fingers into the holy-water font. As the water dripped from my fingertips, I lifted them to my face and touched my nose, cheek, and lips with my now-blessed fingers and circled the area until my fingers were dry.

*   *   *

That afternoon, I called my parents, my brothers, and my closest friends, and told them the news. I was ready. It was time. I made a conscious decision to paint an optimistic picture to everyone. Yes, the tumor was malignant, but all indications were that it had been caught early and that everything was going to be okay. But Rob, my brother closest in age and who I had spent the most time with growing up, had become my closest confidant. We shared with one another what best friends share—our fears and our aspirations, our successes and our failures. Rob was smart enough to know that cancer was cancer. He must have sensed an undercurrent of anxiety or dejection in my voice.

"You're a Leo, Terence," he told me. "You've always been incredibly strong, and this will be no exception. The way you're handling this is so admirable. Most people would be a wreck if they had even a benign tumor on their face."

His words made me realize that I could downplay the situation only so far, even if it did make it much easier to talk to people. I thought that if I was calm about it, maybe everyone else could be too. But Rob was emotional and believed emotions had their place. "It's okay to be angry Terry, it's okay to cry. I know you're going to be okay too, but don't dismiss this like you would a cold. I'm here to help you in any way I can." I was so lucky to have Rob as my brother.

But I knew I couldn't have coped with telling everyone in person, so I subconsciously chose to call because I knew how hard it would have been to handle the silent reactions—the averted eyes, the suppressed gasps—that would have spoken louder than words. Maybe calling was the easy way out, but it was my choice to make.

*　　*　　*

Within a few days, the reality that I had cancer started to sink in. But it didn't sink in very deeply, at least not at that point. I assumed that the worst was already behind me. After all, both Kernan and his assistant had said they had caught my cancer in the early stages. Besides, Kernan hadn't seemed too concerned, so I really didn't believe that my case was that serious. I knew I was going to be okay.

I thought about being cancer-free five years down the road, because I had always heard that the five-year mark was considered the true sign of a cure. My cancer was localized, which meant that if the follow-up surgery biopsy showed that the margins around the site of the original tumor were cancer-free, I was probably cured.

It wasn't until much later that I would begin to learn about the other risks I was facing. For example, my cancer could spread to my lungs, although this was less likely if the tumor had been completely removed from the original site early.

*   *   *

The follow-up surgery was scheduled for February 21, 1985, a month into the spring semester. In late fall, before my biopsy, I had signed up for eighteen units for the spring semester, a heavy load given that most students took between twelve and fifteen units a semester. I had decided to load up because I didn't want to have to take more than fifteen units a semester during my senior year. I also planned to continue working at least two days a week at the insurance company where my father worked.

I had always believed, and still do, that the busier you are, the more you get done and the more productive you'll be with your time. One possible problem with my heavy class load though, was that spring semester was supposed to be so much fun, with deck parties on Thursday afternoons, exchanges with sororities on Thursday nights, and whole blizzards of parties all weekend. And as the weather improved, there would be more and more distractions. But I wasn't that worried. After all, I had survived my first five semesters at Cal just fine.

So as the semester began I went to as many parties as ever, and I continued working out regularly, just as I had always done. I wasn't trying to forget my problems; I simply wanted to continue living the way I always had. I wasn't going to let the cancer make any difference. But maybe I wanted to be so busy that I wouldn't have time to think about my cancer. I pondered that very little, deciding to relish in my life as a student while I could.

*   *   *

Because my tumor was malignant, Kernan felt that it was outside the scope of his practice as an Ear, Nose & Throat (ENT) specialist, so he referred me to an oncologist at the UCSF Medical Center. I felt relieved when he suggested the referral because I had never felt completely comfortable with him since the day he had had so much trouble even telling me my diagnosis, but I would also have been at a loss about how to go about finding another doctor.

The oncologist, Mark Cravens, was a focused, intense man of about forty-five who was in great physical condition. He worked twelve hours a day seven days a week and still managed to look like an athlete. Apparently he ran or played basketball just about every day.

He had little time for chitchat, but we did share an interest in sports, and before long he began heckling me about Cal football every time I saw him. He had gone to medical school at the University of Iowa, and their team had been so strong for so many years that there wasn't much for me to heckle him back about.

He didn't give me much chance to ask questions about the procedure, but his obvious confidence made me feel I didn't need to. I was convinced that he knew what had to be done. When he told me that the procedure would be very simple, he spoke with such conviction that I was sure everything would go just fine.

I could have looked around for another doctor, but I didn't want to. Cravens's credentials were impeccable, and everyone I talked with who knew of him said that he was the best in his field. People also told me that the UCSF Medical Center was one of the best places to be if you had a serious medical problem, let alone a rare condition that only a university would have the resources to research.

I knew that I could lick my cancer; I just needed a qualified surgeon to help me achieve that goal. Maybe I was being naive, but I felt that whether a disease was cured or not had far more to do with the patient than with the doctor. I had always believed in the concept of "mind over matter," and I wasn't about to stop now.

I still think that western medicine, which focuses almost exclusively on physical treatments for diseases, has much to learn from eastern approaches that emphasize mental, emotional, and spiritual aspects of illness. Obviously, both approaches work in some circumstances and fail in others, but I believe that the trend over the past ten or fifteen years toward what's now becoming known as "complementary medicine," which combines both approaches, is a positive one.

I would also like to see more research on how patients' attitudes affect medical outcomes, because I'm convinced that attitudes are crucial to the processes of disease and healing. In his book *Love, Medicine and Miracles*, cancer specialist Bernie Siegel documents the lives of his cancer patients and suggests that their mental attitudes played a far more important role in their recovery than did traditional medicine. I hoped that my attitude would remain positive as I prepared for whatever else lay ahead.

*   *   *

Cravens didn't seem too concerned about my case because he hadn't rushed to put it on the schedule. On February 20, the night before the surgery, I kept to my usual routine and studied in the library a couple of hours. Then I drove out to my parents' home in Walnut Creek. I hoped to get a quiet night's sleep away from all the constant activity at the fraternity, but I also subconsciously felt the need to be with my parents, to feel like I was being taken care of and protected from life's evil and pains. As I lay awake in the bed I had slept in all through high school, I again prayed for strength, for a successful surgery, and a quick healing and recovery. I also prayed that Cravens would eradicate the cancer once and for all.

The next morning, I checked in at the medical center at 6:00 a.m. for my 7:00 a.m. surgery. After I completed the paperwork, I was sent to pre-op, where I met with the anesthesiologist, who described the risks of general anesthesia. He also asked me about my medical history and if I had any known allergies.

＊　　＊　　＊

That morning's procedure with Cravens was my first "real" surgery. I didn't count the biopsy as a "real" surgery because I had had only a local anesthetic. For the first time, I was going under general anesthetic. My mother, who had undergone several surgeries, had told me about some of the possible side effects of the anesthesia. But she said there was nothing to worry about because I wouldn't feel anything until I woke up. She was right. All I remembered before I went under was the anesthesiologist giving me a shot of Valium.

When I awoke after the surgery, my throat was very sore. I was groggy but didn't feel too bad. A few minutes later, I was wheeled from the recovery room to my private room, where my parents were waiting. I wasn't really hungry, but it was after two in the afternoon and I hadn't eaten since the night before, so when the nurse came in and asked if I needed anything, I thought I should ask for some food.

"Would you like anything in particular?"

"I guess a regular lunch tray."

She said that lunches had been delivered more than two hours earlier but that she would see what she could do. Cravens must have written "normal diet" in my chart, because minutes later she brought me a regular lunch tray with a roast-beef sandwich, an apple, Jell-O, milk, and coffee.

"Terry," Mom said, "Maybe you should stick to the Jell-O. The sandwich might upset your stomach."

"I feel fine," I said, and took a big bite of the sandwich.

Mothers are usually right, and this time was no exception. I got through about half the sandwich when out of nowhere I started feeling more nauseated than I had ever felt in my life. A moment later, I threw up all over the bed.

Mom pressed the call button, and within seconds the nurse hurried in to clean up the bed and me. My dad, who didn't seem fazed at all, cheerfully grabbed the other half of my sandwich and the apple. I knew that Mom felt bad for me, but that didn't keep her from appropriating my coffee.

"It'll save me the trip down to the cafeteria," she told me.

Mom and Dad were doing just fine with my lunch tray, but I decided to wait a bit longer before trying to put anything else into my stomach.

*   *   *

My confidence in Cravens continued to rise when I was able to see how delicately, carefully and precisely he had handled the incisions, because I ended up with almost no scarring.

Although he had had to make incisions in my palate and along the right ala of my nose (the ala is the "wing" of the nose, or the tissue that encircles the outside of each nostril), he had placed the sutures right along the crease between the ala and my cheek, thus avoiding any scarring. He had also removed some muscle from my right cheek but had reconstructed the area by moving a bit of surrounding muscle tissue to fill in the gaps left by the removal of the tumor.

He told me that once the incision healed, no one would be able to tell that I had had surgery. My prognosis looked good. Based on the pathology examinations that had been carried out during the surgery itself, all the margins around my tumor were clean. It appeared that the surgery had been a success from both a medical and a cosmetic standpoint.

*   *   *

I stayed in the hospital only overnight, but it seemed much longer. Even though my stay was so short, the idle time alone in my room really got to me, and I started feeling sorry for the other patients and for anyone who had to stay in a hospital for any period of time. Later on, I would learn what it really was like to be one of those "other" patients.

I was excited to get back to the Zete House. I figured I'd be a big hero for a day or two, with everyone asking me questions and looking at me in awe because of what I had gone through.

"Oh, it was no big deal," I would say, hoping for some home-baked cookies from some of my girlfriends and maybe even an extra hug or two.

But my scar was so tiny that most of my friends didn't even realize that I'd had surgery. I didn't have any bruises to give it away either, not even a black eye. But I didn't know then how easy it was for surgeons to operate right next to the eye without causing any bruising. I thought that Cravens was a genius because I walked out of the hospital with almost no visible evidence of my surgery.

*　　*　　*

By the time I went to my postoperative office visit with Cravens, I was already back into my school routine. It was after football season, so he didn't have much to heckle me about.

"First, let's get rid of those sutures," he said. "Everything looks really good, and pathology confirmed that all the margins are clean. We got all that ugly stuff out of you."

"Will I need any other treatment?" I asked, hoping desperately that the answer would be no. At the back of my mind was the preconceived notion that cancer patients usually underwent radiation or chemotherapy and lost all their hair.

Cravens reassured me. "Not at this stage. Surgery is the primary treatment for the type of tumor you had. We're sure we got it all, so all we need to do is keep an eye on you. We'll schedule you for a CT scan every other month or so, but I don't see any reason for concern."

I was ecstatic! He was telling me the cancer was gone! Then I started wondering whether he was telling me everything, but I decided not to ask too many questions. If he didn't seem concerned, why should I be? Besides, I wasn't into worrying because

I believed that, even when it was hard to avoid, it accomplished nothing positive.

I left Cravens's office thinking that for the rest of the spring semester my worries would be just like my classmates' and friends'—the next midterm exam, the next term paper, the economics problem set, and those half dozen books and course readers that had to be read somehow. These worries seemed insignificant compared to the life-and-death concerns that had been on my mind for the past several months.

I told myself that I should be enjoying every day, and to hell with it if I didn't feel like going to the library to study every night. Before my cancer, I would have felt guilty and forced myself to study no matter how I felt. Now, I was determined to stay busy and focus on achieving the goals I set for myself, but not at the expense of not enjoying each day.

CHAPTER THREE

College With My Eyes Closed

Spring semester turned out to be great in all respects. Although I was taking eighteen units, working sixteen hours a week, and attending most of our parties, I still maintained my 3.0 grade point average. Okay, so I wasn't at the head of my class, but I was involved in so many other things besides my courses.

Though I hadn't changed much as a person as a result of the cancer I did find myself focusing on appreciating each day and thanking God that I was alive each morning when I woke up. I promised myself that I would do something each day that made me happy. It might be simply going for a run or looking through albums at a record store, but I resolved that regardless of how busy I was or how much work I had to do, I would take time each day to do something I enjoyed and to take control of my life.

I also found that I was actually happier than I had ever been before. I had learned that there was much more to life than the day-to-day, and realized that I had taken so much for granted in the past. Now I found myself appreciating each sunrise, each sunset, the clouds in the sky, and the trees and the grass that landscaped the hills and meadows. I also learned to appreciate all the people who were in my life as friends and loved ones.

*   *   *

I was looking forward to summer, primarily because I'd had such a busy spring. I had gotten a new job in a downtown San Francisco law firm, and I planned to start the Monday after the end of finals week. I didn't want to take a break after finals because I needed the money and I was actually excited about the opportunity to begin learning what lawyers actually did day-in and day-out. Many of my friends were also working downtown, so we planned to meet after work at places like Schroeder's or Millie's or even the Royal Exchange for a few beers.

That summer I spent a lot of weekends in Berkeley because a couple of my friends were living at the Zete House. Sometimes a group of us would all go out to the local bars and basically do the same things we did during the school year, which was to drink beer and talk about girls and sports.

During the summer, Berkeley turned into a small town. At the end of each spring semester about 20,000 students disappeared from the campus and the town, which made it a nice place to be in a lot of ways. The pace was much slower, and the almost-deserted campus was tranquil. Some weekends, I would just walk across campus and appreciate its stillness and openness. I noticed things I had never noticed before, like the beautiful eucalyptus trees that towered along the pathway that led from Moffitt Library to the Earth Sciences Building. Perhaps I was noticing those things because I wasn't rushing to make it to class, or perhaps it was because my mind wasn't so cluttered with graphs and charts from my economics classes.

But I wondered if I would even have taken those walks if I hadn't had cancer. I think that my illness had taught me that I needed to take the time to see the beautiful things that were all around me, literally in my own backyard.

*   *   *

Before I knew it, summer was over and I was starting my senior year. Back to rushing across campus to make it to class on time. So much for those relaxing strolls, at least for a while, but I was excited about the coming year. All of a sudden I was one of the old-timers, one of the guys the freshmen would call the "older guys."

It was time to start thinking about a career. Most of my fraternity buddies, who came from more money than I did, were planning trips to Europe after they graduated. They would either spend the summer abroad or travel until their money ran out.

I, on the other hand, was starting to think about revising my resume, writing cover letters, and gearing up for a serious job search, even though I wasn't too clear about what I wanted to do. Traveling to Europe or Australia sounded appealing, but I didn't let myself dwell on the idea. Money was tight, and I had just applied for a third government student loan of $2500 to cover my tuition and rent.

I planned to work even more hours during my senior year even though I had received a couple of thousand dollars in scholarship money to supplement my student loans. I knew that by the time I graduated I'd be lucky to have $500 to my name. But it didn't really bother me that I couldn't join my buddies in Europe, because I knew that someday I'd get there.

I already had 90.5 credits toward graduation and I needed 120 to graduate, so I was right on schedule. I signed up for sixteen units in the fall, with the idea that I could coast through my final semester by taking only the remaining 13.5 units. I was feeling very confident and was proud that I was actually on schedule to graduate in four years.

* * *

In the mid-eighties, it seemed as if most students at Cal were taking longer than four years to finish, but graduating in four years was a goal that I had set for myself the day I got accepted to Cal. My three older brothers had all graduated in four years, and I knew they would give me a hard time if I didn't. Besides, I was ready to move on. I was actually getting tired of hanging around the Zete House and partying every night. I had had my fun; now it was time to seek out and meet some new challenges.

I was even planning to take some business and computer classes if I could get into them. I wanted to be able to show prospective employers that I had some business background because I had been told that liberal arts majors often had trouble finding jobs. Employers were generally looking for graduates with business, economics, engineering, or similar degrees.

As a political science major, I had taken many liberal arts classes but no business courses, so I applied for an accounting class, an investment class, and a computer programming course. The business classes were over-enrolled, as they always were, so I settled for the programming class.

* * *

When classes began, so did the parties, and even though I was tired of them, they were hard to resist. By the end of the first week, I was already a week behind in all my classes. This seemed to happen every semester, but like most of my friends, I figured that studying could wait but the parties couldn't.

* * *

The fall semester looked as if it was going to be the same as usual. The first week went something like this:

On Monday, we made sure to attend our classes. We had to

attend class to insure we got our class enrollment cards, even if admissions showed you were registered for the course. If you weren't present the first week, someone else would claim your spot. Oftentimes, you'd find you weren't even assured enrollment in any courses, so you had to hope others would drop out so you could take their spot. This was a classic case of learning the lesson about persistence. It did and still does pay off. That night was our official first brotherhood for the fraternity pledges, and like most frats we ordered that they guzzle lots of beer. The first brotherhood always confirmed who the big drinkers would be and who the lightweights would be.

On the first Tuesday of every semester, we hosted a party called the "Zete Zoo," one of the biggest parties of the semester in the Greek system at Cal. I got to see a lot of people I hadn't seen all summer. It lasted until about two in the morning. People left behind an incredible litter of cups, kegs, and bottles, but that was what the pledges were for. They had to have the whole house spotless by eleven the next morning. The main drawback to the Zoo was that I had to go to my classes the next morning or risk losing my enrollment.

By Wednesday, I was trying to figure how I could get to all my courses on time, given that I had to keep crisscrossing the campus but had only ten minutes to do it. Wednesday evening was a lot like Monday evening except that we let up a bit on the pledges. Even though none of us had done much studying the first two nights, we still went out to one of the local bars, as it was still the 'get reacquainted period'. One favorite was the Kingfish, a classic dive in Oakland that had probably been around for forty years. It looked like a tumbledown shack, but inside it was bigger than it looked and quite cozy. The ceilings were low and the walls were literally plastered with old photos of Cal greats in football, rugby, water polo, crew, and just about every other sport, interspersed with autographed photos of Don Shula, Pete Rose, and dozens of other sports celebrities.

Thursday's were traditionally, though unofficially, the start of the weekend and the biggest party night on campus.

During my first three years at Cal, I had learned to schedule a light class load on Fridays because it was hard to get motivated after Thursday-night parties. That semester, all my classes met on Mondays, Tuesdays, and Thursdays, which allowed me to work all day on Wednesdays and Fridays at the law firm.

That meant getting up at six-thirty to get into downtown San Francisco, but I was twenty-one and seemed to have an endless supply of energy. When I got back, I went out to play an hour or so of three-on-three basketball followed by an evening of drinking beer and watching baseball with some buddies.

*　　*　　*

That semester started out great. Granted, I had to study and write papers, and I always worked part-time, but it didn't seem all that tough at the time, maybe because my time was my own. I could set my own schedule and my own priorities, and I was as free as I had ever been.

But that freedom wouldn't last forever. In one afternoon, those carefree days would come to an abrupt end and I would find myself in a grueling fight to save my own life.

CHAPTER FOUR

Positive Thinking

During the six months after my surgery, the awareness that I had had "cancer" gradually receded to the back of my mind. Cravens had told me that every cell of the tumor had been removed. As far as I was concerned, I was cured.

Although that wake-up call had made me more aware of how much I took for granted, as the months passed I gradually lost touch with my insights about how fragile life was. By the time the fall semester was underway, I was back in the same rut I had been in before my illness. I gradually stopped doing the special "something for me" each day that I had promised myself I would do.

By the third week of the semester, my class routine was set. I knew that I couldn't afford to put off studying any longer. Some of my fraternity brothers wouldn't study at all until the night before an exam, and it was common to see guys typing term papers at two in the morning the night before they were due. But during the previous three years, I had learned that I couldn't afford to operate that way, so I was actually fairly disciplined about studying once I made the first step to the library.

* * *

The fall of 1985 was an interesting time to be a political science major. One of my courses was on South African politics and the nation was in turmoil about the events taking place there. Apartheid had to come to an end, but the fact that many U.S. corporations had economic interests in South Africa meant that they were in effect supporting racial separatism. Because the Regents of the University of California had economic interests and investments in South African companies, many of the students and citizens of Berkeley were up in arms. "Divestiture" was a common word heard around campus, and around the country, for that matter.

There was nothing new about the economic ties to South Africa, but it seemed that semester saw more antiapartheid rallies than any other semester. As a result, the awareness and interest in the events in South Africa led many students to the doors of this particular classroom. The fact that this course and my major in Political Science had some context in the real world made me feel like my education was important. I wasn't just going through the motions – I was learning about the history of apartheid which gave me the knowledge to form an educated opinion and take part in shaping the social and economic change that I and many others felt needed to take place.

Despite my fear of computers, I was starting to enjoy my basic programming course as well. At first it was like learning a whole new language, but as the course went on it started to make more sense. I knew that any company I applied to would be looking for candidates with some type of computer background.

About three weeks into the semester, however, I started feeling uneasy. My concentration level waned, and I felt an almost uncontrollable nervousness come over me at times. My cheek and nose had started to bother me, intermittently itching. It wasn't until that Saturday-afternoon nosebleed though, that made me realize I might have a problem again.

*   *   *

As I stared at the small nub of flesh inside my nostril, I said a quick prayer that what I was seeing was only scar tissue. After all, Cravens had found hardened areas in and around my cheek since my surgery, but he had reassured me that they were only scar tissue. My CT scans had all been negative too.

I tried to put it out of my mind because I felt that dwelling on it would only make things worse. I decided to go right back downstairs to the party. Besides, I wanted to reassure my buddies that I was all right. They all knew about my cancer, and I was concerned that Chip might have thought that he had really injured me. Since my surgery, the guys had been extra-cautious when we played basketball or other sports. If anyone happened to hit me in the face, he would stop and say, "God—are you okay, Heals?" I tried to tell them that my face was healed and no more susceptible to damage than theirs, but they still seemed unusually concerned, and I appreciated it.

So I went back down to the party, but I knew in my heart something was wrong even if I didn't want to admit it to myself. There I was, twenty-one years old and in my senior year. Everything going so well. I was young and healthy, wasn't I?

But then I started remembering that both Kernan and Cravens had said that if the cancer had gotten much bigger, or if it ever came back, the resulting surgery might cause some serious scarring or even deformity.

The word "deformity" scared me so much that my thoughts starting running away from me. I found myself almost hoping that if the cancer had come back it would be too late for surgery and that I would die. I felt that I would prefer that to living through the rest of my life being deformed.

My fears only increased the day after the nosebleed, when I began feeling a tingling in my cheek and around my nose. At first, I wasn't completely aware of it, and I found myself rubbing my cheek because it itched so much. But it wasn't the ordinary kind of itch that could be stopped by scratching. It felt as if ants were crawling under my skin. And one day, when I was rubbing the area, I felt another mass, to the right of my nostril, in my cheek area. This time it wasn't pushing on my nose. Nor was it visibly noticeable, as the first tumor had been.

Despite my fear of being deformed, I didn't really want to die, so two days after the nosebleed I put in a call to Cravens's office.

It turned out that he was on vacation for two weeks. When his receptionist asked if I could wait to see him, I felt panicky and told her it was important that I see him as soon as possible. The receptionist put me through to Cravens's nurse, who was very nice and seemed to truly care about my concerns.

"I don't think you should worry too much," she reassured me. "Dr. Cravens will be back in nine days. Besides, I'm sure everything will be okay. Your recent test results were all negative."

She was right, I thought as I hung up the phone. Nevertheless, I felt discouraged and distressed. The only solution was to keep busy, and the busier the better. Unfortunately, my concentration seemed to grow weaker by the day. During the nine days before Cravens returned, whenever I sat in class or tried to study in the library, I kept thinking about my face rather than my studies. Of course, this just heightened my stress level because now I was worrying about both school and cancer. I tried to do things that I knew I could concentrate on, like running or working out or playing basketball. Spending time with other people took my mind off my worries, so I hung out at the fraternity more and also began leaving the library earlier to go and hang out with friends after studying.

I prayed a lot and tried to envision only positive outcomes when I finally saw Cravens. I pictured myself waiting in his office. He would walk in smiling and shake my hand.

"How are those Bears doing, Terry?" he'd ask. Then he would pull up his stool and take a good long look at my face. "So I hear something mysterious is going on here," he would laugh, sensing that I was feeling stressed. "Well," he would finally say, "everything looks great to me. What you have is a little buildup of scar tissue. Generally, that stuff will itch a little, but it'll eventually subside, and six months from now you probably won't even feel it."

"Do you think I need a CT scan?" I would ask.

He would shake his head. "Not just yet. Why don't we plan on seeing each other in another couple of months when it's time for your next regularly scheduled scan?"

I envisioned these kinds of scenarios several times a day. I felt caught between two attitudes. I was hoping for the best and trying to think positively, but at the same time I was also trying to be realistic and to prepare myself for the worst because I knew that if things went bad, I had better be prepared to deal with them.

I was due to see Cravens on a Monday morning, the first day he would be back. That Saturday night, a group of us went barhopping in downtown San Francisco to celebrate one of our fraternity brothers' 21st birthday. We got back to the Zete House about two-thirty in the morning, but went on celebrating until almost dawn thanks to the kegs we kept in the television room.

I awoke the next morning to thoughts of my nose and cheek. "Shit!" I thought to myself. I had hoped that I'd been dreaming, but I wasn't. I felt empty and lonely, as if I had been dropped off out in the middle of nowhere and had to find my way home on my own. I was scared. The party was over, literally, and the next day I would see Cravens.

*   *   *

Though I was eager to get checked out, I was also in denial, almost wishing that Cravens would be out of town longer so I wouldn't have to see him just yet. The more I thought about my symptoms, the more convinced I was that the cancer had recurred. I was afraid to think about how Cravens might react. Would his eyes widen and his head jerk backward in shock? Or would he just chuckle and tell me that there was nothing to worry about?

I didn't know how I was going to get through the day. I had never been this nervous before a doctor's appointment. I paced back and forth across my room. I started sweating. I felt like just getting on a plane and flying away somewhere, but the realistic part of me knew that I had a responsibility to myself and to everyone who loved me. I wasn't worried about dying, but I wasn't ready for more surgery and more discomfort. I had too many things I wanted and needed to do. For one thing, midterms were the following week, and I was pretty far behind in my studies.

I kept vacillating back and forth between two opposite ideas, first that the cancer had come back and second that what I was feeling in my face couldn't be anything serious. After all, Cravens had cut everything out and the margins had been clean. But ten minutes later I would be back to wondering whether it was cancer again.

Finally I decided that the best thing to do would be to go study at Boalt Law Library, which was right across the street from the Zete House and stayed open until midnight. I read and took notes until eleven-thirty before I called it quits. When I returned to the fraternity television room, I found a bunch of the guys playing Mexicali, a dice game that often involved a lot of beer guzzling in a short space of time. It was another way to keep my mind off my appointment with Cravens the next day, so I hung around for about twenty minutes, drank a couple of beers, and then headed off to bed.

CHAPTER FIVE

Brutal Reality

The next morning was business as usual. I got up and attended classes until noon, came back to the house for a quick lunch, and headed back across campus for my one o'clock class. My appointment with Cravens was scheduled for three o'clock, so I would have plenty of time, or so I thought.

I usually drove my car to the BART station and left it there whenever I was heading into the city because San Francisco's public transportation system was so much more convenient than trying to drive into the city, but given my time constraints that day, I opted to drive all the way to UCSF. My aunt Ange had been nice enough to give me her 1963 Ford Falcon when she decided it was no longer safe for her to be driving, so I was grateful I had the option to drive when I needed to. But when I went to get my car, I discovered that it was blocked. I ran to the key rack where people were supposed to leave their keys if they were blocking someone else but found that the person blocking me had either forgotten to leave his key or, more realistically, had just been lazy or inconsiderate. I had to round up several guys to lift and drag the car out of the way. This cost me about fifteen minutes, and I was feeling just a bit pissed off, not to mention that I was uptight anyway.

*   *   *

I raced into Cravens's office with butterflies in my stomach, and not just because I was late. The receptionist was not concerned that I was late and showed me into one of the examining rooms. Unlike many examining rooms, Cravens's were furnished with dental-type chairs rather than examining tables, most likely because it was easier to examine head and neck ailments when patients were sitting upright.

A moment later, Cravens came in wearing his usual uniform, a worn blue blazer, gray slacks, and striped tie.

"How's everything, Terry?" he asked.

I didn't want to waste any time. I wasn't feeling like myself nor did I want to shoot the shit. "I have a few concerns," I said. "I'm having some weird sensations in my cheek, and I found a clump of tissue inside of my nose that just cropped up."

"Let's take a look." I had learned by now that his manner was always calm, as if he wanted to avoid alarming me. He pulled up a stool, perched on it, and felt my cheek. Then he probed my nostril with his cold, metal instrument.

"This stuff sure showed up out of the blue," he said. "We need to get you scheduled for a CT scan either this afternoon or tomorrow morning. And we'll schedule a biopsy as soon as we can after that. In fact, I'm meeting with the Tumor Board next week and I would like you to be there so that the whole team can take a look at you." His mind moved so fast, I was in shock.

"Even before I have the scan and the biopsy?" I asked. "It sounds as if you're pretty sure this is a recurrence, right?"

The worst-case scenario was becoming reality.

"Well, I really don't know. But we'll have the results of the biopsy by then anyway, and we might as well get you scheduled for the Tumor Board just in case."

I knew that he was trying not to alarm me while at the same time letting me know that something might not be right. I appreciated his cautious, but businesslike manner. I didn't want any bedside manner, any pats on the shoulder, any reassuring "You'll be okay" comments. I didn't want anyone feeling sorry for me. I knew that this was a bad situation, but I also understood that now was the time to move, to take action and make decisions. And because of that, I wanted to get more out of Cravens about what he actually thought about my condition. After all, it was my life that we were talking about.

So I decided to prod him and asked, "Do you think it could be scar tissue, or is it a tumor?"

"I always said that fibrosarcomas behave in strange ways," he replied, "and I think that's what we're seeing here. Based on the speed with which this mass developed, I seriously doubt that it's scar tissue, but we can't rule anything out until you get your scan and we actually go in and excise the area."

Although I had thought I was prepared for whatever he might tell me, I was still jolted by his response. It was clear that he thought my tumor was back. The roller-coaster ride was about to begin.

My first reaction was anger. Just six weeks earlier, he had sent me a letter saying that everything seemed to be under control. How could everything change so suddenly? I was so pissed off that I felt like punching a hole in the wall. I left the office in a rage that I tried to hide from Cravens and his staff as best I could. Angry though I was, I had always been a very rational person, and I knew that anger wasn't going to do me much good now. So I stifled the urge to lash out physically or verbally. As soon as I left Cravens's office, I began trying as hard as I could to focus on the positive. If I had allowed these evil cells to invade my body, I told myself, I had the power to expel them as well. I had to focus my energy towards mind control rather than body control, and on positive rather than negative reactions. I couldn't put off this reality. I had to deal with it now.

Fifteen years later, as I write this, I still believe in mind over matter. I have healed a lot in the respect that maybe then I did blame myself a little for getting cancer, wheras a few years after my fight and onward since then I haven't seen the point in blaming myself. It doesn't do me any good. It makes me feel worse about myself, this self-destructing mentality, so I have just decided that what happened happened, and there is no point in harping on what 'might' have been or what 'might' have caused my cancer. I am who I am and am very happy and confident in the person I have developed into over the years.

*   *   *

In spite of UCSF's huge bureaucracy, Cravens's nurse got me scheduled for a CT scan at eight-thirty the next morning. I was amazed. Usually CT scans had to be scheduled about a week in advance. I also realized that his office was treating my case with an urgency that I had never seen before.

Although I had realized that my visit to Cravens probably would turn out to be a brutal reality check, I had also thought that I would come out of it with a decisive diagnosis. Instead, I would have to wait for the next day to get the "real" results.

I didn't want to assume anything. Who knew what the test results would show? I tried not to freak out. Somehow I found it in me to block out the shock. I started thinking that I might have to do something about my midterms if things didn't turn out as I was hoping. I couldn't help thinking that the prognosis didn't look good.

I hoped that I could depend on some of the habits I had developed to help me cope with life's problems and stresses. Studying was therapeutic for me, as was running and lifting weights. These activities all took my mind off whatever was bothering me and let me focus on how I was doing something good for myself. My running and weight lifting programs were always tied to goals that motivated me to work harder and achieve more, but I never felt as if I was obsessed by these activities.

I drove back to the Zete House unsure of what lay ahead and undecided about whether to tell my family and friends until I knew more. I went for a run, thought it over, and decided not to tell anybody anything just yet. My parents had just left for Italy and would be gone for another week or so. I also concluded that there was no point in worrying anybody until I knew something significant and definite. For all I knew, I was jumping to conclusions. But then, why had Cravens decided to move ahead with such urgency?

When I went to dinner that night, I wasn't myself, but no one seemed to notice. Afterwards I went upstairs and talked with John for a while, as we normally did after dinner. He knew I had gone to the doctor's that day. He also noticed my mood, and he asked me how everything had gone.

I decided to tell him exactly what I knew, which wasn't much. He expressed concern but then changed the subject. I was grateful, because he was an incredibly funny person, and within minutes we were both laughing about something else completely. We agreed to study only until about ten and then head off to the Bear's Lair, an on-campus bar.

I tried to study, but I just couldn't forget about what lay ahead. I finished my problem set, though a bit halfheartedly, and headed to the Bear's Lair a little early. That night I wanted to be with friends.

*   *   *

The smell of pancakes and eggs woke me early the next morning, but I knew that I wasn't supposed to eat for four hours before a CT scan. I got to UCSF in plenty of time to fill out all the paperwork. I tried to focus on reading the newspaper while I waited, but I felt nervous. I had already had four or five CT scans over the previous year, and I had hated every one.

When the technicians and nurses were ready for me, I was taken into the pre-exam room for my IV. Getting an IV successfully really depended on how experienced the person was who was sticking the needle in your arm. The older, more experienced nurses had the process down and could usually get the needle into the vein on the first try. But the less experienced nurses sometimes needed two or three jabs to get it in right.

That morning, the nurse poked at my arm five times before she finally said, "I don't know what's wrong with your veins. They're terrible! I'll go find the head nurse."

A few minutes later, the head nurse, a middle-aged African-American woman with a heartwarming smile, walked in.

"Let's not stick you any more than we need to," she said. "Let's get this little bugger in there once and for all."

And she did. She rubbed an alcohol pad across my vein and without any difficulty at all popped the needle right into place. It was all in her technique.

"Why is it sometimes so hard to find a vein?" I asked.

She got a big smile on her face. I could tell immediately that she was happy that I was interested in what she was an expert at. "Sometimes folks get so nervous that their veins recede," she told me. "Or they might be taking medication, so we can run into problems finding a good one."

I was nervous as hell that day, so it was no wonder my veins had receded.

A few minutes later, just before they wheeled me into the scanner, the nurse returned to inject the usual iodine solution that would make any irregular masses in my head show up during the scan. It always looked to me as if they were pumping a good four ounces of the clear liquid into my IV right before they actually rolled me into the scanner.

Unfortunately for me, I always had a terrible reaction to the iodine. When I had my first scan, I started dry heaving the instant the iodine hit my bloodstream. That was why you weren't supposed to eat or drink for at least four hours beforehand. Apparently, the stomach lining reacts to the iodine as if it's a poison and tries to reject it, hence the dry heaving.

My reaction was more severe than most, though. Within three seconds of the injection, I would heave three or four times. Then the feeling would pass, and I would be okay. I still had the metallic taste of the iodine in my mouth, but I no longer felt sick.

The nurses and technicians were always blown away by my reaction, and every time they had the same response. "God!" they would exclaim in bewilderment. "I've never seen anybody react so quickly and violently before!" Then they would ask me if I had ever reacted that way before.

"Every time, like clockwork," I would respond.

I always tried to warn them, but they didn't seem to take me seriously. Then, when I did react, they were so shocked that I would start to wonder whether there was something else wrong with me.

"So other patients don't react the way I do?" I asked that morning.

"Not that I've ever seen," the nurse replied.

Her failure to attempt to reassure me did nothing to make me feel less worried, but I tried to comfort myself by telling myself that my body was so healthy that it was responding this way because it didn't want to let in any poisons. I was better off than most people were, I told myself, because my body was able to tell me immediately whenever anything was wrong.

A few minutes later, they wheeled my gurney down the corridor to the examining room. I knew I could have walked, but it was hospital procedure. Before I was diagnosed with cancer, the only reason I ever went to a hospital was to see someone else, and I had always thought that anyone being pushed around on a gurney had to be seriously injured or very ill. I always felt especially frightened when I saw young people being wheeled down corridors with IVs dangling above them. Now I knew better. I wasn't sick. I felt fine. In fact, I would probably have worked out that afternoon if it hadn't been for the CT scan.

But then I caught myself. I had cancer. I *was* sick.

I never really thought of myself as "sick" before. I didn't feel sick, and if I didn't feel sick, I wasn't really sick, right? That morning marked the first realization that I might be "sick." It hit me just as I was being wheeled into the CT scan room.

I could die. People died from cancer all the time, and many young people that were diagnosed with cancer died too. I knew two top runners from a competing high school that both died within two years of each other. One was only a sophomore in high school when he died. He was an All League runner. One week after he placed in the top five at the league finals he felt weakened and thought he had contracted pneumonia. Within another week he had died, a victim of leukemia. The other died a slower death, but was gone within a year of his diagnosis.

But I wasn't ready to die. I am sure no one is ever really ready to die, so what gave me the sense that I could beat this thing? I pondered that for a moment and decided not to think too much more about it. I was going to win. I was going to live. I just had to deal with some challenges that I was determined I could get through.

After the scan, I felt relieved. Cravens's nurse was supposed to call me that afternoon and tell me when my biopsy would take place. But although that was still hanging over me, I felt happy. Maybe it was because I hated CT scans and now that it was over I felt like celebrating. I was also hungry, and thinking about food usually made me happy. Life really wasn't that bad, I decided, even if I was facing cancer surgery. If I let myself think about the biopsy, maybe my mood would change, but why bring myself down?

'I should be enjoying every moment,' I told myself. Besides, whatever happened, I knew I'd come out of it okay.

I hurried down to the UCSF cafeteria and grabbed two doughnuts and a carton of orange juice to hold me over during the drive to Zim's Restaurant, across from the San Francisco Children's Hospital in Laurel Heights.

I ordered my usual, the Zimburger with mushrooms and cheese, a large fries, and a large strawberry milkshake. For some reason, I always came out of a CT scan craving junk food. As I was powering down the burger, I realized that I was missing one of my political science classes. 'Oh, well', I said to myself, 'eating and enjoying myself is far more important right now.'

I took my time eating and then headed back to Berkeley. Cravens's nurse was supposed to call between one and four o'clock, which meant I would have to blow off the rest of my classes that day. I didn't want anyone else at the Zete House to answer that call and have to take that kind of message for me. For one thing, it would raise all kinds of questions, and for another I couldn't rely on getting an accurate message or, for that matter, getting the message at all.

To save money, I wasn't paying for phone service in my room that semester, so I used the pay phones installed in the Zete House. We had four phones, two downstairs and two upstairs, but only two lines, so each number rang on one phone on each floor. Anywhere from thirty-five to fifty guys had to share the two phone lines. Sometimes, usually right after dinner, both lines would be tied up for an hour at a time. At other times, people would tie up the lines by leaving the phone off the hook, usually a result of forgetting about it after unsuccessfully trying to track someone down to take an incoming call.

When I got back, I decided to hang out with everyone near the upstairs phones while I waited for my call. Talking with the guys was probably the best thing for me at that point anyway. I knew that even if I tried to study, my mind would keep wandering into thoughts about the biopsy and my test results.

As usual, Cravens's office didn't call until almost the end of the afternoon. But at least I got the call. His nurse told me that my biopsy was scheduled for nine o'clock the following Monday morning at Children's Hospital in San Francisco. I thought that was a little eerie because I'd spent so much time across the street at Zim's and had often wondered what that hospital was like. I would know soon enough.

CHAPTER SIX

The Waiting Game

I was surprised that my biopsy had been scheduled so far in advance. It was only Tuesday, which meant that I had six days to wait. But in some ways I also started feeling better because I thought that if Cravens was willing to wait that long, maybe my case wasn't so serious or urgent after all.

During the days that followed, I was able to shelf my thoughts and worries to some extent, and I found that I was able to carry on pretty well. That night, I phoned my brother Rob. He tried not to sound shocked when I told him what was happening. I knew that he seemed to get a lot of satisfaction out of helping people out, me included, so I wasn't surprised when he asked if he could do anything. Because our parents wouldn't be back from Italy until Monday evening, I asked him if he would take me to the hospital, wait for me, and then take me home. I wanted him there because he was also extremely funny—the ideal person to have around if you had to wake up in a hospital.

At the time, he was living at my parents' house and had a flexible work schedule, so I felt okay about asking him, and he agreed to take me and wait for me without hesitation.

Rob had graduated from Cal the year before and was working part-time at a couple of different places. He was still searching for what he wanted to do with his life. What none of us knew at that time was that Rob was struggling with his own battle, one we wouldn't really know he was agonizing over for another five years. He was still the jovial Rob, but sometimes he did seem a little depressed. I just figured he was struggling with career decisions.

*　　*　　*

On Sunday morning, I packed my laundry and some of my schoolwork into the Falcon and drove out to my parents' house. I didn't know if Rob would be around or not, but we had planned to have dinner together that night, so I figured I might as well head out before I ended up wasting half the day bullshitting at the fraternity about what everyone had done the night before. Besides, my parents' house would be quiet and peaceful, and sometimes I needed a break from the fraternity.

When I arrived, the house was empty. I figured that Rob had gone on a bike ride or something, so I put in a load of laundry and headed for the kitchen. Unfortunately, my mother always cleaned out the refrigerator before she and my dad went traveling. Sometimes she would leave frozen pizzas in case one of us came home, and she usually left a supply of fruit. That day was no exception. I grabbed an apple and a banana, spread my books and notes out on the kitchen table, and actually got some good studying done. Every once in a while I would lift my head and spot a deer or two feeding in our backyard.

The house was set at the top of a short hill that had been an almond orchard prior to the ten-house development built in 1976. A remaining almond orchard in back of my parent's house bordered a steep hill spotted with oak trees and tall grass. Several houses stood on the crest of that hill, but beyond them lay miles of open space crisscrossed only with fire and deer trails. It was a beautiful area, rich with oak trees, but pretty barren otherwise. The hills were inhabited with deer, a few turkey vultures, and even a red fox or two. I often hiked or ran the fire trails and seldom saw another person. Despite the fact that I was in Walnut Creek, I felt as if I was miles from everywhere.

My dad and I used to fight about letting the deer feed in our backyard. He kept threatening to put up a fence, but I kept arguing for the deer's rights. I loved watching them, so graceful and beautiful to the eye. My dad, on the other hand, thought only about his lovely flowers, whose buds the quiet creatures kept nipping off. I could understand his point, but I felt that it was prettier to see deer rather than flowers in our own backyard. He could plant flowers in the front yard, I told him.

A few hours later, Rob came back from what must have been about a fifty-mile bike ride, judging by how long he'd been gone. As I was putting away my books and notes, he walked in, sweat dripping from his chin, and went straight for the refrigerator.

"Hey Terence, how are you?" he asked.

He cracked open two beers, handed me one, and we went outside and sat on the deck.

"I'm fine Rob," I responded. I didn't want to dwell on how I was doing so I shifted the conversation to how we should tell Mom and Dad, given that they would be arriving home the night of my biopsy. I had considered calling them in Italy. It wasn't that I wanted to upset them, but no matter when I told them, they would still be upset.

"I think it'd just spoil their vacation," Rob said. "You know Mom. She'd insist on taking the next flight out of Florence. Besides, they'll be home tomorrow night, and nothing serious is going to happen between now and then."

I finally agreed. The biopsy was only a biopsy. Cravens would not be set up to do anything but take the tissue he needed for pathology, nor would he have my consent for any more extensive surgery.

Still, I was feeling nervous, especially about the prospect of waking up and getting the word from Cravens. Would the news be good or bad? Then I realized that I wouldn't know the pathology results right away anyway. It would take at least a couple of days. And that Cravens was such an optimist that when I did wake up all he would tell me would be not to worry. As I always tried to do, I hoped for the best but tried to prepare myself for the worst. Focusing on the positive had a calming effect. I started feeling less anxious and more hungry.

We headed into the kitchen and Rob began fixing dinner. He wanted me to have a good, healthy meal. Rob had a real flair in the kitchen, and I definitely didn't, so I just stood around and kept him company while he prepared his famous spaghetti with zucchini, mushrooms, garlic, olives, cheese, ground meat, and God only knows what spices.

By the time dinner was ready, we were famished. We wolfed down our food without saying anything but how good it all tasted. I probably ate enough to keep me going for a week.

While we cleaned up, we got to talking about backpacking and whether we could get one more trip in before it got too cold. I could tell that Rob wanted to get my mind on something I could look forward to. At the back of my mind the whole time, though, was the feeling that backpacking anytime soon might just be a fantasy.

I wanted to get a good night's sleep, so after watching a little TV, I went to bed around ten. Rob said he would make sure that I was awake by six-thirty, because we had to leave by seven to reach the hospital in time for registration.

Fortunately, I fell asleep right away. It might have been all the carbohydrates in Rob's spaghetti.

*　　*　　*

The following morning, we left the house at seven o'clock sharp and headed into the thick of the Monday-morning commuter traffic. We didn't talk about the biopsy or about what might lie ahead. Instead, we talked about what some of the guys in the Zete House were up to and what some of Rob's old classmates were doing.

We arrived in plenty of time. Rob stayed with me through registration and told me he would be right there when I awoke. He kept cracking jokes to me about "going under" because Cravens was going to use a general anesthetic. On the drive over, we had heard Bruce Springsteen's "I'm Goin' Down" on the radio. I suppose some people might have thought it sounded like a bad omen, but to us it seemed so appropriate that it made both of us laugh. As I headed toward the pre-op area, Rob shouted after me, "You're goin' down, down, down, down."

But as I lay there waiting for the IV to take effect before I went "under," I couldn't get the song out of my head and I began to wonder whether God was warning me that this really might be the end.

The next thing I knew, I was waking up in the recovery room, with the same words running through my head. "I'm goin' down, down, down, down, hey, hey, yeah, I'm goin' down, down . . ."

One of the nurses asked how I was feeling, told me that everything had gone as expected, and gave me some ice to suck on. She said the procedure had taken only forty-five minutes and that I would be released as soon as I recovered from the effects of the anesthetic. I figured that the tissue sample was already on its way to pathology. I didn't see Cravens. By the time I woke up, he had already returned to UCSF.

As soon as I was released, Rob and I headed straight across California Street to Zim's. I enjoyed my usual cheeseburger but started feeling more tense as Rob and I drove back to Walnut Creek. Sure, I was nervous about the biopsy and about being a subject for the "unusual cases" that had to be presented to the Tumor Board, but I was also nervous about having to tell my parents that the cancer might have recurred. How were they going to take the news that I needed to appear before the Tumor Board, and that they needed to be with me?

Cravens had told me that unusual and difficult cases were brought to the board because it was thought that when it came to rare types of tumors, the more opinions the better. Many of the patients were young people who were facing difficult surgical prospects, but the board also saw patients who might benefit from the combined opinions of not only surgeons but also radiation oncologists, ophthalmologists, oral surgeons, and even maxillofacial prosthetics specialists.

I hoped that because I could feel the lump, it meant that I had detected it early enough. I figured that even if this was a recurrence, at least it wasn't hidden, the way so many cancers were. I was sure my case was fairly clear-cut, even if the Tumor Board did want to see me. The possibility that the cancer had extended beyond where I could feel it never entered my mind.

*   *   *

When my parents arrived home that evening, Rob and I were both there to greet them. We tried to act as normal as possible, and I guess we did a pretty good job because they didn't ask if anything was wrong. I didn't have any packing material in my nostril to prevent bleeding, so they wouldn't have seen any evidence of the biopsy procedure. In fact, I probably looked better than before because Cravens had cut away the ivory-colored piece of tissue inside my right nostril as the biopsy sample.

Mom and Dad were in great spirits. They'd had a fantastic time. The food had been great, the weather had been nice, the history had been fascinating, and the shopping had been good. My news was going to be a real downer, so I wanted to try to pick the right moment. After they finished telling us about Italy, they asked us how we were doing.

Rob told them he was fine, but I started feeling so short of breath that I wasn't sure I'd be able to talk.

"I had a bi . . . opsy today." I had trouble choking out the words.

"Today? Why?" Mom asked. "I didn't know there was anything wrong."

I hadn't told her anything about my concerns because I hadn't wanted to alarm her. Besides, it wouldn't have done either of us any good. She would have just worried, as she always did. It could very well have been scar tissue. It still could be. No one knew yet.

"Well, it kind of just came up, so I figured I should just deal with it. All they did was take a small piece of tissue from my nostril. Really, it was no big deal."

"Oh, Terry, I'm so sorry I wasn't here to take you."

She'd gone to every procedure I'd had, and I knew that she felt terrible because she had missed this one.

"Don't worry about it. Rob and I thought it would be better not to call you because you would've wanted to come home early, and we didn't want you to do that. If it had been something more serious, we would've let you know."

"That was thoughtful of you, boys," my dad said, "but I hope you'll never hesitate to call us if you need to."

"I felt like Rob and I could handle it. I just didn't think it was that big of a deal," I reassured them.

"Did you have a CT scan too?" Mom asked.

"Yes. No big deal."

"Yes, it is a big deal. I feel awful that I wasn't there."

I knew that Mom wanted our lives to be perfect. It tore her apart whenever one of us had to struggle with anything. All she wanted was to protect us. Rob and I constantly had to remind her that life was full of twists and turns, and that things were going to happen that none of us could control.

I told her that I was expecting the results the next day and again tried to reassure her and my dad that everything would be okay. But then I had to tell them that Cravens wanted the three of us to meet with the Tumor Board two days later.

"Apparently, he wants them to review my scan and biopsy and to examine me," I told them. "I think he just wants some other opinions."

"Of course we'll go," Mom and Dad chorused.

I was grateful that our family was always my dad's number

one priority. Even though he had just been on vacation for two weeks, he would take Wednesday off too. He didn't need to check in with his boss; he would just make the time.

Fortunately, they seemed to be taking the news the way I had, with some nervousness but without any fear that my situation was serious. I think we all felt at that point that even if I'd had a recurrence, my first episode with cancer hadn't been too bad, and I had only a localized tumor. I felt lucky to have such a supportive family.

We had dinner, watched a little TV, and went to bed. We were all worn out, especially my parents, because they were still on Italian time, nine hours ahead.

* * *

The next morning I got up early and headed back to Berkeley. I needed to go to class because midterms were right around the corner, and at that point I was ill prepared to pass any tests.

After my last class, I decided to visit the Newman Center chapel. I needed to pray, although I felt guilty about wanting to ask God for the favors of good health and favorable pathology results. As I walked across the campus, I wondered why I only paid special visits to church when I needed help. Why couldn't I stop by church to say a few thanks now and then? I knew that my parents prayed often. Why couldn't I follow their example? I supposed that I was no different from anyone else, in that we all get caught up in our lives and tend to pray only when we're facing a major obstacle or illness.

But prayer always seemed to help me. I've sometimes wondered whether God was actually answering my prayers or whether the concentration induced by praying enhanced my mental outlook and created a healthier and more positive attitude that in turn enabled me to get what I was praying for. Maybe collective consciousness is prayer in its truest form. If groups of people think and believe certain things will happen, we can create self-fulfilling prophecies. Honey bees and ants behave with collective consciousness. Everything they do is for the greater good. They all have a specific task and those tasks enable the colony or the hive to create incredibly powerful achievements. Likewise, we as individuals or as groups can put our minds toward overcoming obstacles and finding solutions to challenges that prevent us from moving forward in life. However, I do believe that if we can link prayer and positive thinking, we're more likely to achieve the results we're seeking. I think that if we're depressed and negative while praying, the energy of prayer is wasted. I believe that visualization enables us to direct our mind toward a better life ahead, which is what a healthy mind needs.

I walked into the chapel and dipped all five fingers of my right hand into the holy water. I lifted my fingers to my face, closed my eyes, and gently patted my cheek, my upper lip, my nose, and my right eyelid as if I were pressing the buttons of a telephone keypad. I visualized my fingers as being those of Jesus Christ washing His blessed water over my face. I imagined the droplets permeating my skin and washing any malignant cells into my sinus cavity. I pulled a paper tissue from my pocket and blew my nose. The process was now complete. Any cancerous cells that might have been living in my body were now gone. I was cleansed.

I knelt down in the pew closest to the altar and began to pray. I prayed that the pathology results would be negative and that the new tumor was confined to an area that would cause little if any disfigurement if it needed to be removed. I visualized myself jumping with joy as Cravens told me that the lump was only scar-tissue buildup. I saw myself running in Strawberry Canyon, shooting hoops, and enjoying good times with friends. I was thinking only positive thoughts, and focusing all my energy on how I was going to be healthy and happy.

When I returned to the Zete House, I tried to keep my mind occupied by shooting a few baskets in the courtyard before dinner. I asked around to see if I'd gotten any phone calls, but everyone said no. Of course, Cravens's office could have not left a message, or someone I hadn't talked to could have taken the call. I couldn't be sure. But as five o'clock neared and no call came, I started feeling better. It had to be a good sign. The mass was only scar tissue after all. But then I started wondering, if it was only scar tissue, why hadn't Cravens's office called to tell me that I didn't need to go to the Tumor Board? And finally I told myself that even if it was malignant, it couldn't be that serious if they could wait until the next day to tell me about it.

*　　*　　*

After dinner, I went up to my room to study, but no sooner did I get settled than I heard a loud knock at the door.

"Heals! Phone for you!" one of the pledges shouted.

I hurried to the door and across the hall to the phone, which was dangling off the hook.

"Hello?"

"Hi, honey, its Mom."

"What's going on?" I asked.

"Well, we talked to Cravens and got the news about your biopsy. But don't worry, honey, we'll beat this thing."

My heart stopped and I felt a lump form in my throat. "What are you talking about?" I shouted.

"Well, the mass was malignant again. Didn't you talk to the doctor?"

I flew into a rage. "That's bullshit! Why am I hearing the results from you? Why didn't they call me first?"

"Cravens's office never told me they hadn't gotten through to you. I guess they called us instead to make sure you got the message."

I was furious. I had a million questions, but it was too late in the evening to reach Cravens. And my parents hadn't asked any questions because they thought that I had gotten all the answers already.

"Sorry I blew up, Mom," I apologized. "I didn't mean to take it out on you. I'm not mad at you. You were just caught in the middle."

"Don't worry about it. We'll get all our questions answered in the morning."

My mother never really got angry with anyone. She was better than I was at accepting things the way they were. After a few minutes, I realized that getting upset with Cravens and his staff would probably not be the best tactic. I needed them on my side.

I thanked my mom for calling and we agreed to meet at 10:00 a.m. outside my office in San Francisco where I was working part time. "I'll pray for you, honey," she said. "And I hope you'll do some praying too."

"I was planning on it," I told her.

I went back to my room and lay down on my bed. Fortunately, my roommate had left for the library, so I knew I could have some time alone.

I thought about what was happening. I had cancer *again*. Maybe what I had really was serious. Maybe I would die. The reality started to sink in. I began to cry. I didn't try to stop myself. I gave in to the tears.

CHAPTER SEVEN

The Tumor Board

I scarcely slept at all that night and woke up feeling too nervous to eat breakfast. Because I had no classes that day, and the Tumor Board meeting was scheduled for eleven, it still made sense to get a couple of hours of work in at the law firm first, meet my parents and brother there and head over with them to UCSF.

As I joined the hordes of other commuters heading into San Francisco on BART, I realized that even if I did have cancer, I was still pretty lucky in some ways. Most of the people around me probably had to work full-time and maybe even more to provide for their families. I worked too, but I was on my own, and all I needed was enough money for my tuition, room, board, and a pitcher of beer here and there. Also, I had good medical insurance because of my father's job, and I knew that if I couldn't work, it wouldn't be the end of the world. My family loved me and I could always go home if I had to.

Yes, I thought to myself as I looked around the crowded BART car, I was lucky. What would the mothers and fathers crammed around me do if they got cancer? What would become of their children? How would they pay all the bills?

*　　*　　*

I spent the morning making photocopies of depositions for one of the young attorneys who had been hired out of USF Law School. I'd thought about becoming an attorney. That was why I'd applied for the law-firm job in the first place, to see what it was like.

Just before ten, I told my supervisor that I was heading off to the doctor but would be back by one or one-thirty.

The Tumor Board met on the seventh floor of 400 Parnassus, a building primarily dedicated to doctor's offices and conference rooms. As Mom, Dad, Rob, and I came out of the elevator and headed toward the reception counter, we passed a huge wall of windows that opened up to a panoramic view of Golden Gate Park, downtown San Francisco, and the Golden Gate Bridge. I was awestricken by the vista through the blowing fog that made San Francisco so unique.

I checked in with the woman at the desk, who knew my name when I gave it. My parents, polite souls that they were, asked again if it was all right for them and Rob to stay with me.

"The Tumor Board is an exchange for the family and the doctors, not just for the patient and the doctor," she replied, and escorted all four of us into an examining room.

Moments later, Cravens popped his head around the door.

"Hey," he said, with a big smile on his face, "How's the Healey clan doing?" He had a way of bringing optimism into most situations, an attribute that I found most appealing. He wasn't insincere, either. He just had a charismatic way about him that made people feel good.

He rolled a stool in front of me to sit down. "Let's take a look at you again." He poked at my face a little and then rose and pushed the stool out of the way so he could speak to me and my family.

"In a few minutes, a whole group of doctors will come in one at a time to examine Terry," he explained. "It won't take long.

Then the board will go into conference to discuss all the patients who have come here today. As soon as the conference is over, and it shouldn't last too long, I'll come back and we'll discuss the outcome of the conference and what course of action we feel we should take with Terry's case."

A few minutes later, the first of what turned out to be a total of fifteen doctors popped into the room. After a while, I began to feel like Play-Dough. Every doctor started out by touching and pressing my right cheek, where the mass was most prominent. Then they would palpate the skin all the way up to my tear duct. I started feeling like a lifeless laboratory specimen, and maybe to them I was. There were no questions asked of me. It was almost as if the doctor's were blindfolded, relying on their sense of touch above all else. They didn't want to get to know me, as any level of emotion could impact the scientific conclusions they needed to draw. Many couldn't even make eye contact with me, and it was very apparent to me that this wasn't a doctor-patient or doctor-family exchange. This was truly a lab specimen that they had a limited amount of time to examine before formulating their final observations and conclusions.

The reactions of two of the doctors were particularly terrifying to me. My heart was racing with fear from the moment the entourage began, but these two magnified my fear and made my heart pound so hard it seemed it would explode from my chest.

The first doctor was a middle-aged, intelligent-looking woman radiation oncologist who examined me and immediately began shaking her head back and forth. The message was clearly "not good." I couldn't believe it. Didn't she realize what she was doing? Was that any way to act in front of a patient with cancer?

The second scare came from Dr. Bottoms, the chief of the head and neck surgery department. He was actually Cravens's superior, a big, powerful man of great experience and respect. Like the others, he pressed and massaged my cheek tissue, but he then did something different.

"Follow my hand with your eyes," he ordered me, moving

his hand right and left and then right and left some more while
he focused on my right eye. He was obviously concerned about
the mass that was bordering the lower shelf of my right eye. I had
felt that the mass was indeed close to my inside tear duct, but
hadn't drawn any conclusions about what that meant. Then, like
the female doctor, he shook his head.

A shock went through my entire body, and I immediately
began to feel that he had made a decision about my prospects
right there. I hated him. I felt like lunging at him and shouting,
"I'm okay! I feel fine! There's nothing wrong with me, you asshole!"
But I was too polite, too reserved, and too rational. I somehow
understood that he and the other doctors weren't there to talk to
me, console me, or tell me their opinions. They were there to
examine me, discuss my case among themselves, and go on to
the next item of business.

After the doctors had finished examining all the patients,
they disappeared into the conference room down the hall, and
we waited in the examining room.

*   *   *

We waited, and waited . . . and waited. And then we waited
some more, for more than an hour. I thought about calling work,
but I figured that the second I left to make the call, Cravens
would come looking for me. And I had already learned that patients had to be prepared to wait endlessly for doctors but were
never supposed to make doctors wait.

Then I started getting hungry, but the longer I waited the
more nervous I got, and that made me lose my appetite. I later
realized that the only thing worse than waiting was learning the
truth about my condition.

*   *   *

At last the door opened and Cravens came in.

"I'm sorry for the delay," he said. "Most of the other cases today were more straightforward than Terry's, and most of the time was spent on his case."

My heart sunk. I tried to focus on what Cravens was saying.

"We also had some differing opinions, and that kept the discussion going on longer than usual. So, here's our diagnosis." As usual, Dr. Cravens did not beat around the bush and this time was no exception.

"Terry, this is a very serious situation. You may lose half of your nose, your columella—the tissue between your nostrils—half of your upper lip, and possibly your right eye."

I almost collapsed in shock.

My heart was thudding so hard that I thought that everyone had to have heard it. My mother and I stared at each other in disbelief. How could this tiny cancer have suddenly turned into a horrific and possibly disfiguring and life-threatening disease that was going to change my life, and my family's, forever?

Cravens gave us several moments to begin to let the news sink in and then added, "We need to schedule surgery right away, and you'll probably need a course of radiation therapy as well."

I was lost in confusion and terror. What in hell had happened to me? Only a few months ago, I'd been in the clear. Now my whole life was falling apart. I'd been religious about seeing the doctor and having the CT scans. How could the tumor have come back with such a vengeance? Then I remembered what Cravens had told me several months earlier: "Fibrosarcomas behave in strange ways."

After telling us that his office would schedule the surgery for as soon as possible, Cravens asked if we had questions. We were all in such shock that none of us knew what questions to ask yet. I was numb, like the frozen lab specimen I had felt like earlier during the examination.

"We'll do everything we can to cure you," he said. "I'll stay

in touch. Hang in there . . . And now, if you'll excuse me . . ."
He left, closing the door silently behind him.

*   *   *

I was so horrified that I was close to tears. Suddenly, I started
feeling nauseated. I jumped up and ran out of the room toward
the men's room. Fortunately, I'd noticed the restroom signs when
we arrived. I shoved the door open. Fortunately, the restroom
was empty and I made it to the toilet in the one and only stall
before I began dry heaving. But because I hadn't eaten in so
long, I couldn't bring anything up. Finally the wave of nausea
subsided.

I sat down on the toilet and began to cry out of sadness and
terror. I cried for myself. I cried even more when I thought about
my mother and father and brothers. I didn't want to put my family through this. I couldn't bear to think about looking at my
mother and seeing the pain and fear in her eyes. It wasn't fair.

After a while, Rob came in looking for me.

"Are you okay?" I could hear the love and concern in his
voice, and it made me want to start crying even harder, but I
tried to get a grip on myself.

"Yeah," I answered. "I'll be right out. Can you wait for me
outside?" I desperately wanted him to leave me alone so I could
pull myself together.

I wiped the tears away, went to the sink, and splashed cold
water on my face.

Keep your head up. I told myself. Stay tough. But when I
thought about seeing Mom, Dad, and Rob again, I just hoped I'd
be able to look at them without breaking down again.

When I came out of the restroom, only Rob was waiting. "I
have your jacket," he said. "Mom and Dad went to get the car.
We'll meet them in front of the building."

"Okay," I said with great relief. Facing just Rob for the moment would be a lot easier.

"You okay?" he asked.

"Yeah. I'll be all right. I'm just a little shocked."

"I was too. I don't think we had any idea it'd come to this. But don't worry, you'll be okay. I'm behind you every step of the way."

As we rounded the corner, one of the doctors from the Tumor Board stopped me.

"Can we talk for a moment?" he asked.

Dr. Tom Zaring, a maxillofacial prosthetics specialist who made dentures and prosthetic devices for cancer patients, was one of the most down-to-earth doctors you could ever hope to meet. I could tell right away that he had a great bedside manner.

He mentioned that he and Cravens thought that I might lose some of my teeth. 'Great, one more thing I'm going to lose,' I thought.

My teeth were close to perfect. They were straight, and I'd never worn braces or even had a cavity. Now I was facing the possibility of needing dentures? What else was going to happen?

Zaring explained that he wanted to take impressions of my teeth and mouth before my surgery so that he would be able to make a prosthetic if necessary. He asked me to come by his office any time the following afternoon. I was even more impressed; he was the first doctor I'd met who was willing to work around *my* schedule. As Rob and I said goodbye to him and headed toward the elevators, I suddenly felt better. The doctors really did care. Maybe Zaring would become a real ally and friend.

Moments later, the frightening thoughts began returning, and I told myself to take a deep breath. As I breathed in deeply and exhaled, it was strange to feel so healthy but know that I was so sick, all at the same time.

We walked outside and into a cool, brisk wind, a common weather condition since the UCSF medical center campus sits at the peak of the hill above Haight and Ashbury Streets. The brisk air felt refreshing on my clammy face. I looked across the street, out above UCSF's Moffitt Hospital to the forested hill of eucalyp-

tus trees behind it and realized once again, as I had so many
months earlier during and after my first bout with my cancer, that
I should appreciate everything and not take anything for granted.

I might lose my right eye.

The fear struck me as I gazed at the eucalyptus trees. What
would that be like? I began thinking about practical things such
as driving. Would the State of California even give me a driver's
license if I had only one eye? How had this happened so suddenly? I had just finished my term as president of my fraternity,
and was at the top of my world.

And what about girls? I had always taken things like dating
girls for granted. And I couldn't remember any girl ever turning
me down. But suppose I ended up with only one eye and half of
my nose removed and portions of my cheek and upper lip removed. I would never get another date. I'd be a total outcast. All
these thoughts and fears had grown up in my mind during the
few short moments it took Rob and me to leave the clinic and
jump into my parents' car.

Rob and I buckled our seat belts in silence as my father
tried to maneuver back onto Parnassus Avenue from the curb.

"I'm so sorry," my father said, and broke down in tears.

"It's okay," I said. I hoped that my reassurance would
stop him from saying anything more because his words had
practically brought me to tears, too. I couldn't bear to see
anyone cry right then. My family's sadness would only make
me cry, and I wanted them to think that I was tough, strong,
and confident. I thought that if I could keep a stiff upper lip,
it would be much easier on them. Besides, crying would have
revealed a weakness in me that they had never seen before. I
don't think anyone in my family had seen me cry since I was
a young child.

But I had to keep biting my lip after my father said those
words. I had never seen him cry before. He had always been the
epitome of controlled emotions. He loved me so much and these
events seemed to be tearing him apart. I felt so much more love

for my father than ever before, hearing and feeling his emotions. He had always been so businesslike and pragmatic that I had never known whether he felt anything so deeply. But now it was for certain. My father loved me a great deal.

Sometimes it takes major events and crises in life to discover who someone really is. With those three words, my father and I experienced a first-in-a-lifetime moment that I'll never forget. I saw him as a human being, not just a father figure. His love for me was genuine. And love was what I needed more than anything at that moment—love and prayers.

By now it was mid afternoon. I had told my supervisor that I'd be back, and I was worried about my image if I didn't return to the office. Maybe she would think I was playing hooky, but I just wasn't ready to tell anyone about what I was facing. I couldn't do it. I asked my dad to pull over at the next pay phone.

"Do you think it's okay not to go in?" I asked everyone in the car.

"Honey," my mom said, protecting me as usual, "I think you're more than entitled to take the rest of the day off."

"I don't think I can talk to anyone at work right now." I felt my voice shaking. I could barely talk. "And I don't want to go into any details about the surgery, either."

"Why don't I call?" Rob offered. "I'll just tell them that the meeting didn't go well and that you're not in a position to talk to anyone right now."

I thanked him and told him to have the receptionist relay a message to my supervisor. My father pulled over and Rob jumped out. A few minutes later, he returned with kind of a smirk on his face.

"The receptionist wanted to know what happened. I told her that you have cancer but that I didn't want to go into details over the phone and that you'd call Liz tomorrow. She kept pushing for me to tell her more, and I finally had to say 'No!' It was bizarre." He was giggling as he recounted the story, blown away that someone would have the audacity to ask such questions. He seemed more humored by it than irritated, and God only knew that humor in the place of irritation was what we needed at that moment.

Dad began heading toward the freeway, and for the next several minutes we drove in complete silence. None of us knew what to say.

Finally, I asked my father to turn on the radio.

"Sure. What station?"

He was really catering to me, because I knew how much he hated rock-and-roll, and that was all I really listened to. I asked him to put on KFOG, at 104.5 FM. After a few minutes, the happy, upbeat music began lightening our mood.

"Terry, I just know you're going to get through this okay," my mother said. God, she was great. So positive, and with such a great attitude all the time.

The song on the radio changed, and I heard:

Just a little more time is all we're asking for
'Cause just a little more time could open closing doors
Just a little uncertainty can bring you down
And nobody wants to know you now
And nobody wants to show you how
So if you're lost and on your own
You can never surrender

The singer was talking right to me. I couldn't believe it. Who was he?

We were heading east across the Oakland-Bay Bridge. The sky was clear over the bay, and the view in all directions was spectacular. The blue water and the trees ahead of us on Treasure Island made me realize how lucky I was to be alive. As I heard the words repeat over and over again, I started smiling.

You can never surrender

Someone had to be watching over me. This was too much of a coincidence.

"Listen to this song! Listen to the words!" I shouted to everyone. "I guess I *am* supposed to fight this thing!"

Suddenly I felt better. In the one minute that the song had been playing, the darkness looming over me lifted and I felt optimistic and full of hope and confidence again. Fortunately, the song was one that you could hear and understand the lyrics. I listened on.

> *And if your path won't lead you home*
> *You can never surrender*
> *And when the night is cold and dark*
> *You can see, you can see light*

Yes, yes, things were going to get better, I thought to myself.

> *'Cause no one can take away your right*
> *To fight and to never surrender*

When the song ended, the disc jockey came on and announced, "That was Corey Hart and 'Never Surrender.'"

I knew that "Never Surrender" had just become my theme song, the song I would play if I ever started feeling down about my prognosis or my condition.

As we headed across Treasure Island toward Oakland, we all found ourselves smiling. Corey Hart had given us a new lease on life.

CHAPTER EIGHT

Anticipation

Though I was feeling a little better by the time we got home, I still had no appetite. Everyone else was hungry. None of us had had a chance to get any lunch. It was 4:30, and the consensus was to just have an early dinner. I knew my mother would try to force me to eat even though I would resist it. She would insist that I eat because, despite not being hungry, my body needed nutrients now more than ever. And she was right. She was my loving Mom. She wanted to insure I was as strong as I could be.

I sat down at the table with Mom, Dad and Rob, and moved the food around in circles for awhile before bringing the fork up to my mouth. Without my mother having to insist, I forced myself to eat as much as I could.

After dinner I realized that my clothes, my toothbrush, and even my car were all still back at the fraternity. My books were there too, but I wasn't too concerned about them just yet.

I would need a ride over to the Zete House the next day. 'How could I face those guys right now?' I asked myself.

*　　*　　*

I realized that very few of my fraternity brothers really knew what was going on. I had kept my cancer scare pretty hush-hush around the fraternity house. John was probably the only one who knew I was going to the Tumor Board.

I would just grab my stuff and go. Hopefully no one would even see me. I would just haul everything down the back staircase to my car in the parking lot. Maybe I could get away without having to tell anybody. I wasn't ready to talk to friends about this yet.

*   *   *

The next day was a tough one. I woke up and was instantly reminded of what lied ahead of me. I was hoping it was only a dream, once again, but everything was very clear and vivid in my mind. There was no doubt the Tumor Board meeting was for real. I had to deal with it.

I was supposed to hear from Dr. Cravens that afternoon. He said he would call with a scheduled surgery date. Given the proximity of the tumor to my eye and other vital tissues, Dr. Cravens was trying to schedule the surgery as soon as possible. He indicated to us at the Tumor Board that he would call my parents' house by Thursday afternoon with a date and time.

I figured I could head over to Berkeley and get some of my essentials in the morning so that I would be available when the doctor called in the afternoon. I didn't want to hear this news secondhand like I had the pathology results.

Rob was nice enough to take me over to the Zete House. He planned to drop me off, since I was going to drive my own car home.

*   *   *

When I walked into the house, I said a few hello's to various guys and worked my way upstairs to my room. I hadn't been gone that long, so no one would have really wondered where I was anyway. I was hoping I wouldn't run into John. I thought it would be easier to call him from home. My fear was that if I told him in person, the shock on his face would only make my despair greater. I was facing a horrible ordeal ahead, and I didn't want my worries exacerbated by someone else's reaction. I felt bad, because John was my friend and he deserved to hear the news from me. But John was an emotional guy and I wasn't ready to see him cry nor was I ready to cry in front of him. I was a twenty-one year old fraternity guy. I was supposed to be tough.

I did not run into John, nor anyone else that questioned what I was doing or where I was going with my big bag of clothes. I had successfully escaped.

On the drive home, I tried to take notice of the beautiful trees and golden hills that surround the east bay. It was a pretty area and I was very fortunate to live there. I was so lucky to be able to run and bike in those hills. I had two arms and two legs. I had so much to be thankful for. I reminded myself that my odyssey ahead could be much worse. Yes, I would be disfigured, but I would still have at least partial sight and all the rest of my senses. I would still have my arms and legs. I could still live in the same world when I returned from this, couldn't I? I wondered and I hoped.

I pondered this question for a while. I loved to exercise. Using my arms and legs meant being able to hike, run, bike ride, play basketball and lift weights. I was very independent. I liked people, but I was always able to keep myself occupied when I was alone. I would still be able to do all the things everybody else did, whether by myself or with others. I was lucky. But was I really just counseling myself? Could I really live in the same world when I was through with this? I wondered. Dr. Cravens had told me that he'd get my face back to where it was before the surgery. He told me that at the Tumor Board. My face could be rebuilt.

I wasn't thinking at that stage that reconstruction was going to dominate years of my life. I guess I thought reconstruction was like the plastic surgery stories you heard about on television or read about in *People* magazine. Amazing things could be done to those people in Hollywood. I knew so little, really.

I was so concerned about getting home in time for my doctor's phone call in the afternoon that I rushed to get home by 1:00 p.m. I had some lunch, but my nerves really made it difficult for me to eat. Nevertheless, as my mother preached, I had to keep up my strength. After eating, I couldn't decide what to do. I had to stay in the house so that I wouldn't miss the call. I didn't want to study or work on the essays that would soon be due. I really didn't feel like I could concentrate on anything, so as the minutes slowly passed by, each one seemed like an hour.

At 4:00 I still hadn't heard from the doctor, so I decided to call him myself. On top of the fact that he hadn't called me, I had come up with dozens of questions while I waited for the call. I needed some answers. I called his office at UCSF and was told he was in his car, heading from one hospital to the other. The receptionist knew who I was and went ahead and gave me his car phone number.

I dialed the number and Dr. Cravens answered.

"Hello," he said.

"Hi. Dr. Cravens, this is Terry Healey."

"Hi Terry. Can I call you right back? It will be just a few minutes, okay?"

"Sure. Do you have my number?" I asked.

"I sure do. I'll call you in just a few minutes."

"Thanks," I said, and hung up the phone.

In less than one minute the phone rang. "Hello," I said into the receiver.

"Hey, this is your doctor, and guess what? You're gonna die!" came the reply from the other end of the line.

My heart started palpitating, and before I had a chance to respond, the phone went dead. "Oh my God," I thought to myself. "This couldn't be Dr. Cravens," I said to myself as I stood holding the phone in silence. Somehow though, it sounded very much like him.

"Honey, what happened?" my mother wanted to know, as she could tell the telephone call had ended. "What is going on?"

I actually started to cry. I could not believe what I just heard. But who else but my doctor could it have been? I started to walk into the family room, shaking in fear and confusion. Who in the hell was *my* doctor? That could not have been him. Is he just tired of dealing with all my calls and questions? Is he fed up with me or is he just psychotic? One million more questions started running through my head.

Then I started to panic. I was supposed to have surgery right away, but there was no way I was going under the knife with that man in charge. Oh my God. I had to start all over again. I would have to find another doctor at another hospital. Could this all be a joke? Would somebody play that kind of a joke? The coincidence was too great, wasn't it?

I told my mother, father and Rob what had happened. I knew it couldn't have been Dr. Cravens, but who the hell could it have been, and who would have known that I was facing a life-threatening illness?

I was overly sensitive to everything at that point. It was probably the one day in my life that I couldn't take a joke. The timing couldn't have been worse.

"What do I do?" I asked them. "Should I call him back? I have to know what is going on," I said, holding back tears.

My father encouraged me to call him. He was convinced someone had intercepted our call and was playing games. "Terry, Dr. Cravens is a very professional Doctor. But call him and tell him to report what just happened," he instructed me.

I agreed. I dialed his car phone again, nervously. Now he'll really hate me, I thought. My father was right. Why should I wait the few minutes for his return call? Screw it! If he was the one who called, I needed to know now. I was vulnerable and I didn't have the time or the energy for this nonsense.

"Hello," Dr. Cravens answered.

"Dr. Cravens, it's Terry again."

"I'm sorry, Terry, but I have been tied up on the other line."

Fortunately, I chose not to be confrontational. "Well, right after I hung up with you I got a very disturbing call. Somebody called me from a car phone, told me he was my doctor, and said I was going to die."

"Oh, Terry I am so sorry. Someone must have intercepted the call." (This was the early days of car phones and security was not very good). "I will call my cellular carrier and report it right away. Don't you worry. We're a team and we're going to beat this thing together." He then proceeded to tell me that surgery was scheduled for Monday at 7:00 a.m.. He gave me some other details, answered my questions, and apologized again for the disturbing call I had received.

When I put the phone down, I felt like a total fool. I had just made a total idiot of myself. I was twenty-one years old and someone had tricked me into believing that my doctor would say a horrible thing like "you're gonna die!" I guess it seemed after hearing the news from the Tumor Board, anything was possible.

As a kid, I had made many a crank phone call. And I did some other mean things, but I know I could never have been that evil. My only hope now was that I wouldn't get more calls from whomever it was that made the first one.

I've never forgotten about that crank call. The coincidences were just too great. The guy posed as my doctor, he called me right back as my doctor had promised, and he told me I was going to die, which I suppose was a possibility at the time. I thought about Sybil, the woman with sixteen personalities. What if my doctor really did have a second personality? What if he did make that call? He could have made it and forgotten. Stranger things have happened. I guess I read too much. I really didn't think my doctor would do something like that, but on that day of my life I didn't know what was up and what was down. I was a nervous mess. I just wanted the surgery to be done. I didn't know how I was going to get through the next few days and I certainly didn't need someone to make jokes about my life. I never did follow up with my doctor on the incident. I just wanted to move forward and forget about it. Bringing it back up would only renew my anger.

*   *   *

The time had come to talk to friends about what I would be facing. I didn't want to make the calls, but I didn't want to become a hermit about it either. I called John, Tyler and my friend Dave, who lived in Spokane, Washington. Tyler and Dave had been friends of mine since the seventh grade. My mother had already informed Steve and Brian, my other two brothers, and that had taken some of the pressure off and helped ease some of my anguish.

I played down the seriousness of my condition. I told them that I had a recurrence and that I would be having surgery Monday morning. When you tell someone that you've had a recurrence, and the surgery is scheduled only four days in advance, the reaction is expected to be one of shock and concern. My friends were smart enough to understand that it had to be serious if surgery was being scheduled that quickly. Nevertheless, I told them that the doctor was confident he could remove the tumor and I reminded them that my tumor was localized and hadn't spread to any other part of my body. That was always the question—had it spread?

I agreed to meet John, Tyler and some other friends at the Kingfish on Saturday night for beers, dice and shuffleboard. I told them I wanted to hang out Friday night at home to get some good rest.

I knew I would run into a lot of people I knew at the Kingfish and I was a little concerned that word might travel about my condition. I didn't want to talk to people about my prognosis at that point. I honestly didn't know what lied ahead. If people had questions, I didn't really have the answers for them. I just wanted to go and have a good time with my friends before the surgery.

Spending time with my friends would get my mind off of myself. I needed to clear my head of what had been occupying it for the last seventy-two hours. I knew my close friends wouldn't ask me any more questions on Saturday night. They wanted me to have a good time too.

I figured I would only be in the hospital a few days or so after the surgery, so I assumed I would be back to school and everyday life within a week or so. I made sure my friends knew that this was not a send off party. What I was facing probably wouldn't be that big of a deal. I was tough. I could handle it. At least that was what I wanted people to think.

Saturday night was a lot of fun. The plan was to meet at 9:00. When I showed up there were a lot of people inside the bar. It was loud. People were already shouting and dice cups were already smashing across the Formica tables. A crowded and raucous group at the Kingfish always made for a better time. My friend Kerri Conrad was there, which made me happy. She was probably the coolest girl I had ever met. She also could hang out with the guys better than any girl I knew. She could drink as many beers as a lot of guys could and she even chewed tobacco. Kind of gross you might say, but it was refreshing to know a Kappa Kappa Gamma sorority girl who was relaxed enough and secure enough with herself that she really didn't care what people thought of her. The only twist to our relationship was that she had had a crush on me for the last two years and for some reason I just wasn't that romantically attracted to her. She was cute, but she was just too much like one of the guys.

I looked around the bar and noticed a couple of pretty girls. As I admired them, I realized that I was judging people based on their looks. How could I still think that way, knowing I was going to be disfigured? I decided not to ponder that question too deeply that night. I wanted to have some fun.

Kerri and I had gone to parties together. In fact, just recently I had been her date to the Kappa formal. We danced until 4:30 in the morning, but I just couldn't get romantic with her, though

I came very close on many occasions. I guess she was such a good friend that I was afraid that would all change if I ever crossed the line.

I spent a couple hours that night at 'the Fish' talking to Kerri and, I must say, she had the greatest, most upbeat personality you could ask for. She was in my face, giving me a hard time about not pounding my beer fast enough. She was a true friend and a real delight to be with. Even though there had been some tension between us that I kind of faulted myself for, she never changed the way she acted around me. She was the same no matter what. I probably led her on a few times and that was wrong, but I guess I was never really sure if I wanted to date her or not. Interestingly, Kerri and I went through some real ups and downs as friends after that night at the Kingfish, and one night we did get a little romantic. But that was much later.

Kerri had heard about my recurrence through John. I wasn't sure at that time whether Kerri was having a hard time dealing with the fact that I had cancer. She made sure I knew she had been informed before I got a chance to tell her. When I first sat down with her she patted my shoulder and said with a big smile, "Healey, you're gonna be fine. Let's go play quarters." Was she being a friend trying to get my mind off of what lied ahead or was she just the kind of person that couldn't talk about it or deal with it? I didn't ask myself that question at the time, but later I would discover that she really couldn't deal with my illness. It was upsetting to realize that because a friend didn't know how to deal with my situation, she would just plain ignore it and me. As the saying goes, you learn who your friends are. Though the whole episode put a crimp in our relationship, I forgave her when I was old enough to realize that none of us were mature enough to know how to deal with a friend or loved one who became ill. This was a new experience for most of my friends as well as for myself. My friends crowded around me at the table the whole night. There wasn't any dialogue about my cancer. But there were lots of pats on the back and a few toasts to "a successful surgery."

I had a great time at the Kingfish and I thought of Kerri that night only as a great friend for making the effort to make the night fun and well worthwhile.

* * *

Sunday I went to church with my parents and we all prayed that the surgery would be a success. I visualized waking up to the doctor's smile and positive words, "we got it all and you look just like you did before the surgery."

My mother had invited Father Fitzgerald from the Newman Center in Berkeley for dinner that night. After dinner he wanted to offer me the blessing for the sick. I was appreciative to have that opportunity. As he performed the ritual in our living room, I visualized Father Fitzgerald being Jesus Christ and as his hands touched me I imagined being touched by Jesus Christ. I truly felt blessed that night. Despite my feeling of contentment, sleeping was still a real struggle. I tossed and turned as I thought about the next morning. I was nervous because I really didn't know what to expect. The one thing the doctor did tell me was that he expected the surgery to be about a four-hour procedure. I knew I could handle that.

Once I went off to sleep, I must have slept pretty well, because the alarm jolted me out of a deep slumber. I usually wake up less than five minutes before the alarm goes off. My mind tells my body when it's time. However, I feel like I have slept better when the alarm wakes me up, so I was happy to be awakened by the alarm on this morning.

My father liked to allow about two hours to get to the San Francisco Airport when it really took no more than one hour. Well, his plan was for two hours to get to UCSF too. He had spent his working life in the insurance business and I guess the concept of risk had taught him that there was always a possibility there would be a terrible accident or a freeway closure due to roadwork. What bothered me on this morning though was that if

I was early I might have to sit around and twiddle my thumbs and that would make me even more nervous about the procedure. I would rather just walk into the hospital and be escorted into pre-op so I wouldn't have time to really think too much about what was ahead of me.

We arrived early as expected, but fortunately, upon checking in, the medical staff was ready to get started with me. Medical professionals are not like postal workers, that's for sure. Far from being nine-to-fivers, at 6:30 in the morning the nurses and technicians acted as if their first cup of coffee had been three hours ago; maybe it had been.

The staff was aware of the seriousness of the procedure and knew that my parents were at the hospital with me. When the anesthesiologist had my IV ready and was rolling me toward the operating room, he told a nurse to check with my parents to see if they wanted to see me one last time before surgery. Within a couple of minutes my mother was at my side, smiling as usual. Though I knew she was a little stressed, she had a way of exuding an incredible amount of positive energy. To this day, I am still amazed by that quality she possesses. She kissed me, wished me well and said "Go get em. I'll be right here waiting for you when you wake up."

The transformation of my life was about to begin.

CHAPTER NINE

Making Me 'Streetable'

Waking up in the recovery room from surgery was a terrifying experience, and one that was different from any recovery room experience I had before. Never had I felt so beaten up. There was still a tube lodged in my throat, as if the recovery room nursing staff hadn't expected my awakening so soon. I could barely breathe, my throat hurt so badly. I was awake, but I couldn't yet open my eyes. I tried desperately to open my eyes, but a thick, gooey salve was preventing me from doing so. My heart started racing. Did I lose an eye? Why couldn't I open my eyes?

I immediately began thinking of the movie "Johnny Got His Gun". "Johnny Got His Gun" was an anti-war film about a soldier in World War I whose life is saved after being blown up by a mine. The even more horrible part is that he is doomed to live a life on a hospital bed with no sight, no sound, no arms and no legs, but with a mind as healthy as it ever was. He suffers the worst kind of imprisonment and no one else knows how healthy his mind really is.

I began calling for help, as Johnny so helplessly tried to do. "Help. Help. Help," I repeated, unsure whether I was in a room by myself or in a recovery room ward. I thought I must have been in a room by myself or I would have heard nurses and medical staff conversing or using the instruments they needed to do their jobs. Getting no response, I was even more frightened. Unfortunately, calling for help was hard to do because I still had a tube down my throat. Probably what could be heard was not "help", nor at the decibel level you'd expect. but something like "elllp", a barely audible chirp. I called out again and again, but it hurt too much so I gave up.

It felt like an eternity as I lay there waiting for someone to help me. It probably was only a few minutes, but every second felt like an hour.

Finally, I heard voices approaching me. "Hey, lazy, it's about time you woke up," someone said. "How are you feeling Terry?" she asked.

I replied as best I could. "Iddy!" I said, meaning to say "Shitty!"

"Let me get this tube out of your throat, and then I'll give you some ice to suck on," the nurse said.

Thank god, I thought to myself. My mouth was so dry. I knew from experience that they wouldn't let me drink water right away or I would throw it up.

"Hold on," the nurse uttered as she juggled the equipment in front of her. "This will take just one second. Here we go." She yanked the tube out of my throat, and it felt like it was ripping the skin all the way out. Then it was over. My throat was sore, but I felt a thousand times better. I still couldn't see, but I was feeling a lot more alert all of a sudden.

"What's on my eyes?" I asked, almost afraid to hear the answer.

"Oh, it's just Duolube. It's a sterile eye lubricating ointment. The doctor uses it to reduce the dryness in your eyes." She started blotting my eyes with a wet pad, and before I could even ask if I still had my eye, I could feel the pressure from her fingers on my right eyeball. Suddenly I was opening both of my eyes and peering right at my nurse.

"They saved my eyes!" I jubilantly shouted at her. I was ecstatic. Losing my eye had become my greatest fear.

"They sure did," the nurse replied. "And you sure are lucky.

They had to cut right up to the edge of it. But I will let your doctor fill you in on all the details. He should be in to see you in a little while. Go ahead and rest for a while. We will probably keep you in recovery for another couple of hours."

I was thrilled, but as I began to move my head, I felt a tug on the right side of my cheek. I tried to peer down, but all I could see was a long, cylindrical tube running from my chest up to my face. "What's this tube attached to my cheek?" I asked.

"That is what we call a delto-pectoral flap. They had to borrow the tissue from your shoulder to fill in the lost tissue from your cheek. Don't worry. We've seen Dr. Cravens do many of these procedures. The flap is like a living skin graft. In order for the tissue to take on your cheek it needs its original blood supply from your shoulder. It usually takes about two weeks for it to take. Once it takes, they cut the tissue and reattach it to your shoulder. But don't worry. Your doctor will explain everything to you shortly. Try to rest and relax if you can, Terry," she said maternally.

"What the hell?" I was asking myself. "I never was told about a 'flap', was I? What in the hell did they do to me in that operating room?" But I was really too tired to solve these questions now.

I was in and out of sleep for a while after that. I was awakened by my mother's voice. "Hi Terry," she said. I looked up at her to find my brother Rob and my father smiling down at me. "You're a real trooper, honey. Ten and one half-hours of surgery. Can you believe it?"

"What?" I asked. "Ten and a half-hours? God, no wonder I felt so shitty when I woke up. I figured it was four like the doctor told me it would be." My heart started racing again. Why had it taken so long? That was not a good sign. "Do you know why it took so long?" I asked.

"Well, the doctor wanted to be sure the margins were clean. He didn't want to have to go back in there again. He checked in with us every couple of hours. He had to send tissue samples to pathology, wait for the results, and until the tumor cells were gone, he had to stay in there with you. Cravens said you were strong as an ox." I could tell mom was tired.

"What time is it?" I asked.

"It's about 10:30 honey. You didn't wake up until just a little bit ago. But you're gunna make it, by God," she said loudly.

"You didn't have to wait," I uttered. "You guys have had a longer day than me. I have been asleep all day. I'm okay. You should go get some sleep."

Rob had a way of making me feel at ease by describing everything in a humorous way. "When we walked in here, I thought you had a tube hanging from your nose, Terence. But it's skin. You have a big frankfurter hanging off your face. Now all you need is some mustard on there and you have yourself a meal, Terence."

I laughed and thanked them for waiting for me to wake up. I would be in a private room in a couple of hours and I would see them there tomorrow.

Shortly after they left, I heard some nurses enter the recovery room. "Okay, Terence, are you ready to get out of here?" a male nurse asked.

"I'm ready. Take me away," I said. "But is my doctor going to see me tonight?"

"He'll probably see you in the morning. He's been on his feet since 6:30 a.m.. He won't forget about you. Don't you worry."

They were rolling a gurney in next to my bed. "Okay. We're going to lift you onto this gurney. Just relax, it shouldn't hurt." I felt four hands straining to hold me flat as they lifted me onto the gurney.

They rolled me out of the room and into an elevator. Seconds later the elevator door was opening and I was rolling down another hallway. It was very dark. The patients were sleeping. We passed a nurse's station and then made a quick left into my room. I was going to be literally right across from the nurse's station. I was happy about that. It meant I could probably holler for help and at least be heard.

Minutes later a nurse walked just inside my door and stopped. I could see the silhouette of her holding a syringe over her head. The room was black inside, but the light behind her made for a scary but funny scene. If I were more alert, maybe I would have been a little frightened at the sight of someone holding a syringe up in the air at me. "Do you want a shot of morphine?" the female nurse asked me.

"No, I think I'm okay," I replied.

"I'd think twice about that if I were you. You might not feel pain at the moment, but if you don't take this shot, believe me, you're gonna feel it. This shot will keep you feeling comfortable. If I were you, I'd take it. Enjoy life a little. How often does someone offer you a shot of morphine?"

I started laughing. What a cool gal, I thought to myself. She sounded about my age too. "If you say so," I replied.

She walked over to my bed and introduced herself. "I'm Carolyn," she said with a big smile. "You just had a major surgery, but I can tell that you're a stud. You'll do just fine. But let me tell you something. It is in your chart to get a shot every three hours, and if I were you, I'd take every one of them. It is no fun being in the hospital, so make it as comfortable for yourself as possible."

What a great girl, I thought to myself. What more could I ask for in a nurse? As my eyes adjusted to the darkness, I could make out the outline of her face and hair. She had really short, dark hair, a pretty face, and she appeared to be fairly thin. Not bad looking, I thought to myself. Being in the hospital wasn't so bad after all.

Three hours later, I was asking for another morphine shot. It wasn't that I could feel the pain so much, but rather I couldn't get comfortable in the bed and I hadn't slept except for the short period of time after my first morphine shot.

It was difficult to sleep given that different nurses entered my room about every fifteen minutes to check on me and make sure I was laying on my side. I had to lay on my side so as to clean out my lungs of all of the anesthetic. When you lay on your back, it takes longer to eliminate the toxins and the mucous build-up, I was told.

Lying on my side, with a flap of skin attached to my cheek from my shoulder was about as comfortable as standing on my head. I had to tilt my head enough so that I couldn't feel a tug from the stretching tissue. I was also concerned that if I moved ever so slightly, I would rip the sutures out and this tube of flesh would drop limply toward my chest, projecting blood in all directions.

When Carolyn's shift ended at 7:00 a.m. I thanked her for encouraging me to take the morphine shots. It relaxed me enough to get a little bit of sleep and that was better than lying in an uncomfortable hospital bed staring out the door and unable to move in any direction.

As the light entered through my windows from the morning sun, I breathed a sigh of relief. Thank God that night was over. It had seemed like an eternity. I wasn't hungry, but I thought breakfast would give me something to do.

"Will breakfast be here soon?" I asked my new nurse. I was feeling more alert now, and suddenly wishing I had someone to talk to. Just then I felt something foreign inside my mouth. I wondered what had become of my teeth. For the first time I could feel a plate inside of my mouth. My upper front teeth felt somehow different, but I couldn't figure out what the difference really was. I couldn't feel any pain from whatever the doctor had done in my mouth. I actually felt like I could eat. Hey, things weren't so bad, were they?

"Your doctor has indicated on your chart that you shouldn't be eating any real food yet," she replied. "I think he just wants to keep you on the IV drip. I'm not sure how long you'll be on the IV. You should definitely drink plenty of water though."

"You know, I am not really hungry anyway. But I cannot understand why," I said.

"Well, your I.V. is more or less made up of sugar and water. The drip is continuous, and it is intended to keep you from feeling hungry. Some people are on IVs for a long time. Hopefully you'll just be on it for a day or two."

The nurse applied some kind of topical ointment to my face and washed off my flap. She gave me a good looking over and asked if I needed anything else.

I asked only for my dose of morphine when it was time. She said she would be back with it shortly.

As she exited, I heard footsteps and a loud voice from the corner of my doorway excitedly say, "Hey, Terry!" I knew the voice right away, and less than a second later, Dr. Cravens entered my room and walked up next to my bed. "How are you doing partner?" he asked excitedly, full of cheer and all smiles.

"Not bad," I replied, feeling like if I responded negatively, my doctor would think less of me. I wanted him to think of me as someone who was positive all the time.

"Well, we did okay," he said. "I'm sure you have a million questions for me, so I'll just give you the lowdown on what we did and hopefully that will answer most of them."

Dr. Cravens's greatest personal attribute as a doctor was that he maintained complete confidence at all times. He never wavered or showed uncertainty. He was honest, but always positive. He focused on the good, and downplayed the bad. The fact that the surgery ended up being more than twice as long as he had projected never even came up in our discussion. He controlled the replay of events.

Obviously, my concern was that if the surgery was that much longer than planned, quite possibly there had been problems.

Dr. Cravens started by saying that it appeared he had removed all the tumor cells. He was confident that the margins were clean around my eye, and he was enthusiastic that my eye was saved. I guess he was more concerned about my eye and the outcome of the surgery than he had indicated to me before I went under the knife. But what I instantly realized at that moment was that because Dr. Cravens was so optimistic and because he downplayed worse case scenarios, I, as the patient, had been better off. Some might say they would prefer to know the possibilities up front and be aware of what the odds were associated with their type of cancer. I am glad I had a doctor who had a positive attitude, because at that stage in my life, Dr. Cravens was like God to me. He, alone, largely influenced whether I thought good or bad thoughts. When he told me before the surgery, "we're gonna get this thing" I believed him. When he told me it appeared he had removed all the tumor cells, I would have been surprised to hear differently. Dr. Cravens was confident in his abilities, which gave me confidence in his abilities, and that in turn gave me the confidence and positive attitude necessary to fight the disease I faced.

Dr. Cravens then told me that he'd make me "streetable" before I left the hospital and that he'd reconstruct me back to the old Terry before too long.

"What is 'streetable'?" I asked, confused.

"We're gonna get you looking good enough to walk the streets. When the nurses get you up to walk around later today, you can look in the mirror and you'll see what I mean, Terry. Right now you have this flap hanging off your face. But don't you worry. We will need about two weeks before the tissue takes and then we'll remove the excess and get you back to normal."

I had such confidence in Dr. Cravens's abilities that it did not occur to me at that moment that being 'streetable' meant I was very disfigured and that getting me back to normal meant I had a long road of reconstruction ahead of me. If Dr. Cravens said I would be okay, I believed him. I could handle being disfigured temporarily, right? I could act tough for a while and show all my scars to whoever wanted to see them, because it was only temporary, right? I could play that part for a while. Little did I know.

Dr. Cravens told me to keep my right arm at my side and not to raise it for any reason. Likewise, I was to keep the right side of my face at a slight downward angle. This delto-pectoral graft, also known as a Bicangian flap, was sutured to both my face and my chest and a tug in any direction could break the sutures, though it would be unlikely.

A dressing covered the right side of my chest, over my pectoral muscle, protecting the muscle from infection, since all the skin had been moved to my face. Otherwise, raw, red muscle would have been exposed. Another dressing covered my shoulder. Dr. Cravens used a 3" circle of tissue from my shoulder to graft to the right side of my nose and cheek. The dressing was protecting that donor site with another single thickness skin graft from my thigh.

I wasn't even aware of the thigh skin graft until that moment. I pulled back my sheets to expose my leg. A transparent, cellophane-like dressing covered an area about 7" in length by 2 1/2" wide. Through the dressing it looked like a bad raspberry you might get from falling off your bike and colliding with the pavement. I touched it and still felt no pain. Why had I always heard that skin graft donor sites were extremely painful?

Dr. Cravens was off to perform another surgery, so our visit was brief, but informative. He told me he would be back to see me later in the day.

Someone had come by and delivered a newspaper on my tray table, so I picked it up to read. Perhaps because of all the morphine I had had, I couldn't concentrate on the newspaper for the life of me. I read a couple of paragraphs and wondered what I had read, kind of like when you're falling asleep and you try to finish that last page—somehow you get through it, but nothing makes sense and you cannot remember a word you've read. I decided I would be better off watching talk shows and old reruns of "Leave It To Beaver."

Not long after I flicked the television set on, Mom, Dad and Rob arrived. They were all smiles, a very welcome sight. I was already bored and it was only about 8:30 in the morning. The shift nurse after Carloyn left was nothing to write home about. I already missed Carolyn.

Rob and my Mom were more interested than Dad in checking me out, looking at my dressings and examining my flap. Rather than showing shock at what they saw, they both kind of laughed at the collage of bandages, sutures and the flap that hung from my face in the shape of a long hot dog. Their reaction made me feel much better. If they weren't shocked, then it probably wasn't so bad after all. As I would later find out, most people did look at me in shock and disbelief. But my family loved me for who I was, and always would. Their reaction to me was sincere. My appearance in that bed was more humorous to them than it was shocking. Their reaction in turn made me laugh and made me believe that if there was laughter there could be happiness, no matter what I looked like.

But how long would I maintain my positive spirit? How long would I be able to reinforce to myself that life was still very good, and that I had so much to be thankful for? I felt like I could handle it, but comments made over the next couple of weeks in the hospital would begin to make me worry that maybe I should be depressed—maybe I shouldn't be happy. That first day marked my first experience with the "words of wisdom" from a social worker at the hospital, who, to this day, I feel has no business touting her credentials as a social worker for patients.

The social worker entered my room about mid-day while Rob and my Dad were down having lunch in the hospital cafe. A middle-aged woman, plain in dress and attitude, she hinted of trouble immediately.

"Hi, Terry. I'm Rita, the social worker here on staff." She didn't wait for my reply. "I think you'll find that you may need to talk to someone about your condition. I am here to help you with that."

Not being one for psychologists or psychiatrists, I always felt if I needed to talk about something that bothered me, I had my family and friends who supported and understood me. Perhaps I hadn't experienced the problems and difficulties in life that would make me want to reach out to a professional.

"Well, I am doing fine. I don't think I need that right now. I am very confident that my condition will improve," I replied.

"I'm sure you feel that way now, Terry. But believe me, there will be a time when you'll need to talk to someone. You have been through a very traumatic experience. Not only is it about cancer, but a disfiguring cancer too."

I became very angry all at once. I was feeling like my privacy had been invaded. Did I invite this person into my room? How dare she walk in here and tell me how I am suppose to feel. Those were the thoughts boiling in my brain at that moment.

"You know," I said, "I am doing just fine. I didn't have any negative thoughts until you walked in my room."

She sat there next to my mother, emotionless. She had the same expression on her face now as she did when she spoke. It was as if she was lifeless.

She replied finally, "Maybe you're not ready yet. That is okay. But let me assure you—I know from experience that you will need to talk to someone at some point. I just want you to know that I am available to help you."

She never smiled. She never showed any enthusiasm in what she was offering me. She was expressionless. I couldn't believe my eyes. What kind of social worker is this? Was she really supposed to be a counselor for patients on this floor? Couldn't UCSF find someone with a little more spirit? Couldn't they find someone who used a different approach? I wouldn't have been so defensive if she had come in to ask how I was doing, instead of suggesting I needed help. Why wouldn't she try to size me up first before offering her services and suggesting I talk to someone?

One thing was for sure. If and when I ever needed to talk to someone about my situation, I was sure that she would be the last person I would go to.

When she finished speaking, she just sat there, looking at me. No smile, no hopefulness in her face. I started wondering if maybe I was screwed up. Maybe she was right. I shouldn't be happy. I should be sad. I should be hopeless. Maybe I was much worse off than anyone would ever tell me. "BULLSHIT!" I said to myself. No one is going to strip me of my positive attitude and hopefulness.

Finally, my mother stood up and said nicely to Rita. "I think Terry is very tired. I think he needs to take a little nap. Thanks for stopping in." Hint, hint. It was my mother's way of saying, "get out of this room, NOW!"

My mother is such a sweet person. She couldn't say a mean word to anyone. She has a way of making everyone her friend. People like my mother and that is a good thing. The only problem is, people like Rita cannot read the true meaning of her words. Rita would never know that my mother found her invasive and obtrusive. However, my mother had gotten her to exit from the room, and that was all that mattered to me at that moment.

I was almost in tears, I felt so horrible. My mother came to my side and could see and feel the pain in my expression. "Honey, I'm sorry. She was so negative. I don't blame you for saying what you said. But if you do want to talk to someone, your Dad and I would be happy to help you." In other words, they would pay for a shrink.

That made me feel even worse, because that comment made me realize that my parents had already discussed this issue. Was she telling me that I needed or would need help, too? I had to ask myself why I was feeling so positive lying in that bed. I wasn't angry. I wasn't sad. I wasn't scared. I wasn't afraid of going out into the real world. Was something wrong with me? It seemed at that moment that everyone else felt I needed or would need help.

"I don't need a shrink!" I screamed back. "I'm fine. My attitude is great, or at least it was until a couple of minutes ago."

"Okay. I am sorry, Terry. I didn't mean it in a negative way. I meant it in a positive way, but if you don't feel you need to talk to someone, that's okay too," Mom replied.

I guess I was being a little oversensitive at that moment. I was trying to prove my strength and courage. I associated shrinks with problems and negative experiences. I truly felt that my experience, at least at this stage of the game, hadn't been traumatic enough to warrant talking to someone about it. I was fine. I was ready for the next challenge.

"Let's just drop it, okay. I don't need to spend time thinking about things that upset me right now. I need to heal," I said. "But, please do me a favor. Tell the nursing staff that I never want that woman in my room again. She is like the devil. She preys on the weak and vulnerable to make herself feel better about her own miserable life."

My mother didn't really say anything immediately. She wanted me to settle down. She was not used to seeing me upset.

"Well, do you agree with me? Was she evil or is it just me?" I asked.

"You're right, honey. I wouldn't want you talking to her again either. I will tell them that you are doing very well and she doesn't need to spend any more time with you. I'll tell them that we will let them know if we need to talk to Rita. And Terry, I didn't mean to upset you. I don't think you need to go to any shrink either. I was just making the offer to you. I think you're great. And you really look fine too. They'll get you back to Terry."

That was what I needed to hear, because that confirmed what I believed. I was going to be just fine and before long I would look just like before.

*   *   *

I hadn't yet seen myself in the mirror. By exploring the contours of my face lightly with my fingers and from what people had told me, I had concluded that I was very swollen. As a result, looking at myself in the mirror wouldn't mean much anyway. Every day the swelling would go down and I would look better, I assured myself. I also had a flap hanging across my face, which I could feel. Though curious, looking in the mirror would only reflect what I looked like at that moment. I knew my face was going to get better and better. It always did before.

I was wise enough now to know better than to run to the mirror. From my prior surgeries I had learned that it was devastating to see big green sutures poking out of your swollen face, a face that looked like it hid the missing water balloons that only moments ago were ready for launching. When the nurses said I could get up and walk, I would go look at myself. But I reminded myself that everything was temporary. Before I would even be released from this hospital, I was going to have another surgery to remove the flap.

I rested. I slept. I talked. Whenever I woke up that day, my mother would be sitting there with a big smile on her face. She must have just sat there and watched me sleep, and as she saw me begin to awaken, she would make sure the first thing I saw was her smiling and hopeful face. It was the most comforting feeling to know that if anything happened to me as I lay there, my mother would be the first to make sure I was taken care of.

As the afternoon wore on, I knew I would soon be getting a new nurse. I was hoping it would be Carolyn. My wish was granted and this time I would be able to see her in the daylight.

She walked into my room right as her shift started. "Hey Terry. How are ya?" she asked with spunk. She was the complete opposite of the social worker I had encountered only hours before. Carolyn was positive, energetic and good-looking. She carried herself with such confidence. I got a good look at her. Her hair was jet black and her skin, very white. She had on a big black overcoat with pins all over it. She wore bright blue funky earrings. She was a punk rocker, through and through. In the past I had never been attracted to that type, but maybe I was changing. I found everything about her to be sexy.

I introduced her to Rob, Mom and Dad. I could tell instantly that everyone liked her humorous and aggressive style. She wasn't afraid of being herself. Carolyn seemed to get a kick out of shocking people. If they couldn't take it, tough. She made comments like, "Hey Pop (referring to my father) how's your lazy son doing today?" Though my Dad is conservative and polite, he has always admired anyone that has confidence in themselves. My mother pretty much likes anyone who enjoys talking and Carolyn had the gift of gab. Rob liked her because she was an individual who didn't conform.

Carolyn had sized me up right away. That night about 9:00 she walked into my room with a Walkman and some music tapes. "You've probably had enough of the TV by now, so I brought you a little rock-and-roll and a little punk." She guessed I liked rock-and-roll like most twenty-one year old guys and figured she would take a chance and give me some punk music to try out too. What Carolyn gave me was tempered punk and I liked it.

I wondered what Carolyn did for fun. I was sure that she knew how to have a good time. I let my mind wander a little.

I also liked Carolyn because she was thoughtful. She seemed like the kind of nurse that considered the needs of her patients beyond the medical care she was required to give. She wanted me to feel comfortable and at home while I was there. I couldn't stop thinking what it would be like to go home with her after her shift was over.

Every time I saw Carolyn it made me think how wrong the social worker really was. Carolyn treated me as if I was the most normal person in the world. She didn't feel sorry for me nor did she make me feel like there was really anything wrong with me. It made me realize that people who didn't know me could treat me just like my family did—as if nothing traumatic had happened. And more than anything else, that was the way I wanted to be treated. I wouldn't realize until later though that not everyone was like Carolyn. Some people either couldn't hide their feelings or were so curious that they had to rudely ask, "God, what happened to you?"

Probably if Carolyn did act differently toward me, I would still have liked her. Who really knows? But one lesson I did learn from spending time in hospitals was that hospitals could be a very comforting place because most medical professionals have seen or heard about almost every medical condition. Nothing really shocks them anymore. They treat you for the most part like they treat everyone else and never do I remember any of them walking in my room and dropping their jaw in shock as they peered at me. That really didn't start happening until I began life in the outside world again. But I wouldn't re-enter that world for awhile.

My night sleeps were fretful. Trying to get comfortable in a hospital bed when you could only lay on your back with your neck cocked in one direction was a little difficult. I probably was sleeping a lot more than I thought I was, but the nights seemed very long.

I was awakened the next morning at about 7:00 a.m. by an entourage of white coats. I woke up, and staring down at me was about five or six medical people, all fairly young, and one of them was explaining to the others my condition and the details of my procedure.

"Hi, Terry. I'm Dr. Gambel, the chief resident here. At my sides are some of the other residents here who are doing their residency in head and neck surgery," he informed me.

I said hello to all of them and then Dr. Gambel asked if it would be okay for him to show them all the sites affected by my procedure.

I was open to them exploring whatever they wanted, as long as they were careful. I was either a great study for them or I was just part of the daily rounds. I didn't ask, nor did I really care to know.

When Dr. Gambel finished his show and tell, he asked if I was getting everything I needed.

I replied that I was, but decided to ask him when I would get off my I.V. and start eating again.

He flipped through some of his papers and said he would check and let me know. The white coats followed Dr. Gambel out the door. A couple of minutes later Dr. Gambel returned.

"I think you're going to get to eat a little something this morning. You'll be on soft food for awhile, because of all that work that was done in your mouth. I doubt they want you chewing yet, even though your denture is pretty snug in your mouth."

I began pondering what had happened to my mouth. Dr. Cravens had told me that I had lost my two front teeth and the next four teeth to the right of my front teeth. I had never had a cavity in my life. I had never had any kind of dental work, not even braces. My teeth were perfect and all of a sudden I was missing six teeth and about one third of my hard palate. As it turned out, the cancer had spread from my cheek and nasal area into the roof of my mouth, thereby requiring the removal of the six teeth. I wasn't overly concerned about the loss of my teeth, because I knew that dentures were made to look pretty real and I was sure this would be the least of my defects.

It was shocking that I was able to talk exactly as I had before. For that I was thankful, but I was astonished that my mouth never really hurt as a result of all the cutting that took place inside of it. To fill the void in my mouth, I had what they referred to most commonly as an obturator, a denture more or less, that replaced my teeth and all the gums and palate that were now missing.

Chewing was going to be interesting. It would be a new challenge for me, but I had all the time in the world. I wasn't going anywhere for two weeks.

As Dr. Gambel said his good-bye so that he could catch up to his colleagues, a new nurse walked in the door. Her name was Kathleen, and she was one of those women that couldn't wipe the smile off her face. She laughed constantly. I had scored again. Another young, cute nurse, probably twenty-five years old. She informed me it was time for my morphine shot, so I obliged her by rolling partially onto my side, yielding my bare bottom for the

needle to penetrate. The morphine had become part of the proto-
col. I never really asked for it anymore, unless I knew my three
hours were up and Carolyn was my nurse. Asking for the shot
would be an excuse to get Carolyn back in my room.

I enjoyed the morphine. It relaxed me and made staring at
the blank walls actually somewhat enjoyable. I still didn't really
understand why it was being administered to me. I don't really
remember being in much pain at any point. I guess I figured if it
was prescribed, I might as well accept it. Besides, Carolyn had
told me that first night that if I didn't get the shot, I would feel the
pain. That was what the nursing staff was trying to avoid. Their
instructions were to keep me comfortable.

Within seconds of getting the shot, I told Kathleen how
amazed I was that the reaction was so instant. A warm, soothing
and relaxing spell flowed through my body as I spoke to her.
From head to toe, my body melted.

She told me that they wouldn't keep me on this much longer
or I could get addicted. The guy in the room next to me had been
in the hospital two months. He was a paraplegic and had recently gotten in a car accident that was causing all kinds of
complications. She told me he was constantly complaining about
pain and had received so much morphine that he had become
an addict, or was showing the signs of an addict anyway. Two
months after the accident he was still asking for it, but the medical staff had been instructed to keep him off the morphine
regardless of his complaints. Kathleen told me he would throw
things across the room when his morphine was denied. As a result, the nursing staff had to be very careful about who cared for
him.

Kathleen looked at her watch, reminding herself that she
had many more patients to attend to. Moments later a tray was
delivered to my side table. Solid food, at last. Well, solid as solid
can be. On the tray was a bowl of Jell-O and some broth. Better
than nothing. As I started in on it, I realized this wasn't really
"food"—it was what was commonly referred to as a "soft diet"

menu. I would call it a liquid diet, since I really just swallowed everything. I mowed it down in no time flat. I was ecstatic that I finally was eating something. I had started to worry that I was going to lose weight so fast that I would really look like I was sick. You see so many patients on television and in hospitals that look so thin that they appear sick just by that fact alone. I had an appetite and therefore wanted to eat. That morning's breakfast was exciting, and tasted good, but I didn't really get to use my new teeth. Would it hurt to chew? I couldn't wait to start eating real food.

After eating, or slurping, I opened the newspaper and searched for the television listings. At 9:00 was "The Walton's", 10:00 was "Leave it to Beaver", 10:30 was "The Andy Griffith Show", and 11:00 was "Divorce Court". I figured that would be my morning, unless something better came up. I found "The Today Show" as I flipped through the channels, but there was a lack of news, so I half read the paper instead. As I lay there bored, Kathleen walked in again to check on me.

"Do you want to get cleaned up today? Maybe go for a little walk?" she asked.

"That sounds great!" I replied, at once enthused, partially because Kathleen was always full of smiles and seemed like a fun person to be around. She was also pretty cute. I couldn't understand UCSF. I never even expected one pretty nurse. UCSF wasn't a bad place to convalesce at all.

"Why don't we get you out of bed when you're ready. Then I'll walk with you in case you're unsteady or off balance. After that, I'll help you get cleaned up. How does that sound?" Kathleen asked.

Once again, I replied, "That sounds great! I'm ready now."

"Let me check on one other patient. It might take another ten minutes or so, okay?" Kathleen said.

"I'll be here," I replied. She laughed and turned around to exit the room. She had very nice legs. I wondered how she planned to help bathe me.

As she was leaving, my brother Rob and my mother were

arriving. My mother practically collided with Kathleen, and, as is typical with my mother, she never hesitates to start a conversation when she has an opportunity. She proceeded to introduce herself and within moments Kathleen and my mother were like old friends.

It was very important to my mother to know who was caring for me, and when she liked the nurse caring for me, it made her happy to know she could trust his or her care.

Kathleen got a kick out of Rob and suggested he wear the shirt he was wearing that day every day to the hospital—that is if he didn't smell in it, of course. Rob's shirt was white and the graphic on the front was "Mr. Bubble" from the bubble bath product. "Mr. Bubble" had a big happy face and the bubbles all around him were in pink and blue. It was the kind of shirt that made anyone laugh. It was stupid. It was funny. It was hilarious, actually.

I motioned Rob to come toward my bed. I quietly told him that the nurse was going to help bathe me.

"I don't know if she is going to help me in the shower or do it some other way, but I'm kind of stressing about it," I said.

"Why, Terry?"

"Well, I'm pretty attracted to her actually," I replied. "What am I going to do if I get an erection in the shower? How will I ever look her in the eye again?"

"Terry, don't worry. That's not going to happen. And even if it does, she'd understand, and more than that, she'd probably be flattered."

On that note I started fantasizing and quickly developed the framework for a "Penthouse Forum" story. As fast as I was developing my story, I caught myself and brought myself back to reality. I felt guilty for even thinking those thoughts. Kathleen was wholesome, sweet and the kind of girl you would take home to Mom, not to the "Penthouse Forum".

A few minutes later Kathleen walked in, holding towels and shampoo. Finally I would be able to get out of bed and walk around. I realized how lucky I was that I had two healthy legs to walk on. The poor guy next door wasn't going to be able to walk these hallways ever again. I had so much to be thankful for.

Kathleen helped me out of my bed. I was a little shaky at first, but standing for a moment helped me to gain my balance. Kathleen told me that I would have to roll the IV dispenser along with me, because the medical staff wanted to make sure I held down my breakfast before they removed the IV dispenser from my arm. I noticed then that the only thing about me that was sore was my forearm. That IV needle in my forearm was causing the most discomfort of all. I would have thought that would have been the least of my problems, but it seemed the nurses were always pushing on it and changing it. It made me feel like I was in pretty good shape if that was all I could complain about.

I asked if I could look in the mirror before we walked. She helped me into the bathroom, and I paused before I looked up at myself. I took a deep breath and peered out of the tops of my eyes since my head was angled downward from the flap.

Surprisingly, what I saw was somewhat what I expected. Having touched the contours of my face and nose and having heard from the doctors and nurses the details of the procedure, the disfigurement was as described. My nose looked as if half of it was gone. My eye looked okay. My lip was turned up slightly. The flap made me look like the elephant man.

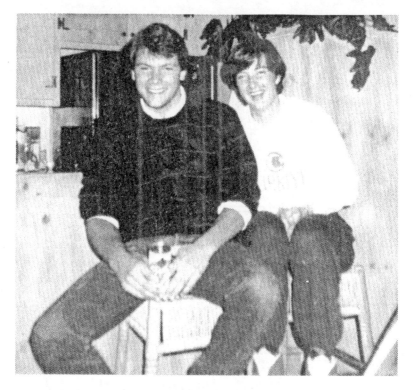

Relaxed and happy before my cancer diagnosis, 1984

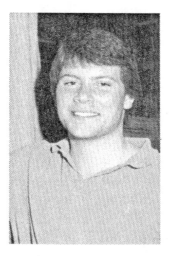

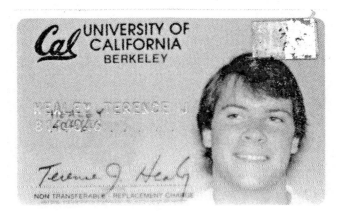

My photo I.D. that showed the initial distortion to my right nostril before I had seen any doctors

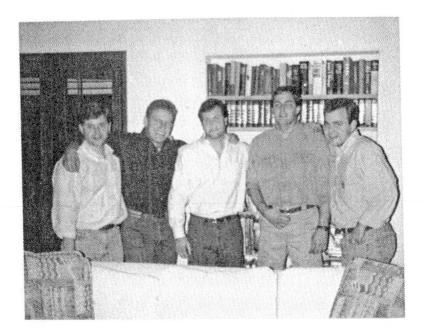

Some of my greatest friends. Standing, left to right: Tyler, Tom, myself, Dave, Cory

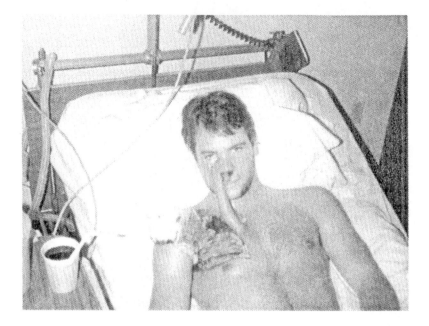

Recovering from the surgery and the initial attempts at reconstruction in October, 1985

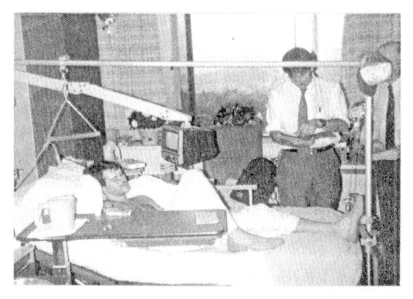

Recovering from follow-up procedure two weeks later

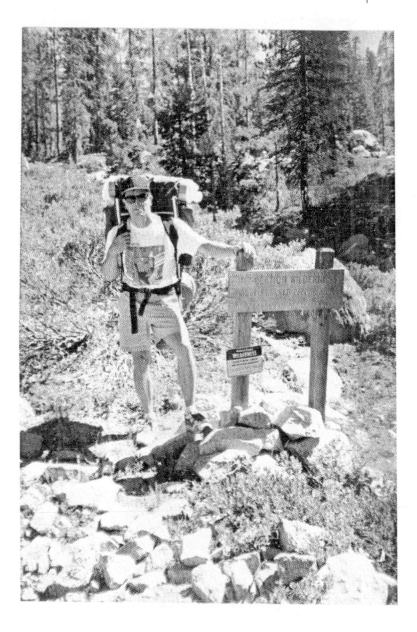

Backpacking in Desolation Wilderness, near Lake Tahoe

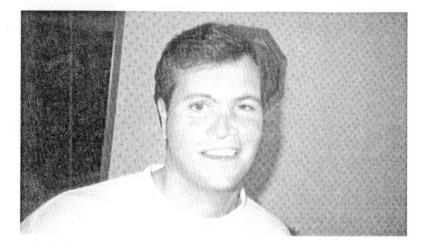

After the last of my reconstruction in 1991

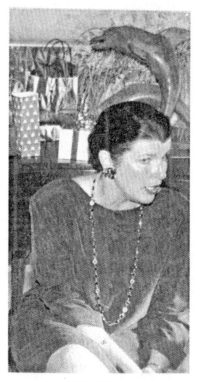

My Mom

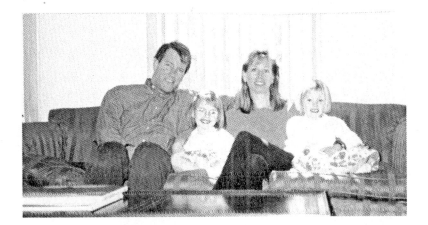

My brother Steve with wife, Ann, and daughters Michelle and Shannon

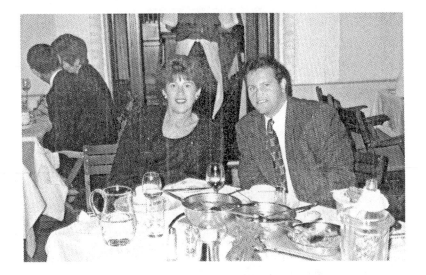

My wife Sue and I in 1995

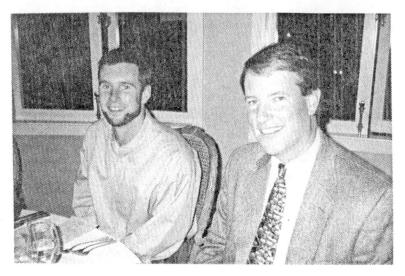

Rob and Steve at Mom's 60th birthday surprise party

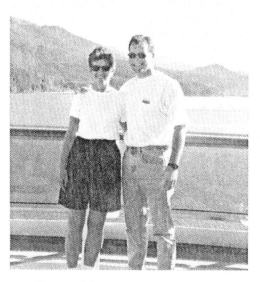

Sue and I on vacation in 1998

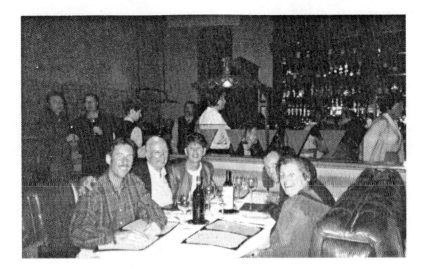

Celebrating Dad's 70ᵗʰ birthday in 2000

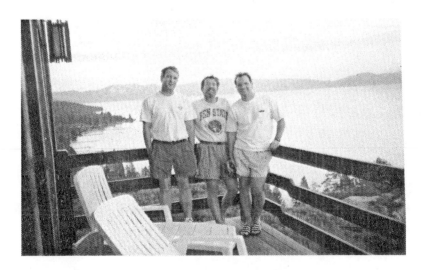

Steve, Brian and I in Lake Tahoe in 2000

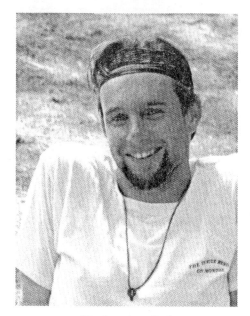

My brother Rob

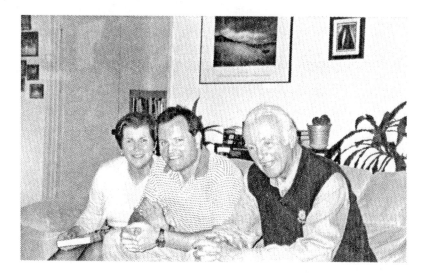

Mom, Dad and I

CHAPTER TEN

Encounters with the Outside World

I realized how serious my condition really was. I concluded that I didn't look like Terry Healey at all anymore.

Kathleen was checking my IV and trying to appear busy without looking at me so that I could familiarize myself with my new face. She must have known this was a critical point in my recovery. She probably had no idea what kind of reaction I would have, but she stood there next to me, regardless. I turned away. Staring any longer wouldn't have helped me. I was ready to go on the walk.

Kathleen reminded me to keep my head down so as not to pull on the flap. She told me not to worry about watching where I was going. She would guide me in the right direction. Rob and Kathleen walked with me a little ways down the hallway and then turned me around.

"Feel okay?" she asked. "Let me know if you feel funny at all."

I replied that everything felt normal. I suggested we walk some more, but Kathleen didn't want me to overdue it, so I conceded. I forced myself not to think about what I had seen in the mirror, as hard as that was to do.

The moment of truth would soon be upon me. The next activity was bathing. Kathleen suggested I take off my gown and try to get myself as clean as I could in the shower without getting any of my dressings wet. She told me she would help me a few minutes later with my face, hair and back.

I asked Rob to stay close by in case I got disoriented or unstable in the shower. Here I was taking a shower, and Mr. Bubble was staring back at me as if I should be in a bathtub. I thought to myself, "Don't you worry Mr. Bubble. When I can take a bath, I will, but right now I have a cute nurse ready to take a shower with me, so I don't think I'll rock the boat right now."

Kathleen knocked on the door. "Everything okay?" she asked. "Pretty good," I said. "Am I not suppose to bend down?"

"No, don't bend down. I will help you with the areas you can't reach," she replied. "Don't be bashful, cause here I come."

I realized Kathleen had probably done this one hundred times and it didn't make her the least bit uncomfortable. It was her job. She probably saw this kind of stuff every day.

As she walked in, she acted exactly how she had before. She wasn't uncomfortable and therefore I was suddenly comfortable about her helping me.

She told me to turn around in the shower and get my back wet. I followed her directions. She hadn't given me much opportunity to hide myself. I stood there as she scrubbed my legs with soap and water. My penis was staring her in the face. She lathered me with soap up to my thighs and stopped. I quickly turned again so that now my back faced her, and I was able to rinse the soap from my legs. She began massaging the bar of soap on my back and then crouched down on her knees and proceeded to lather up the rest of my backside down to my feet. I was beginning to get embarrassed. Now my rear end was practically in front of her face. She left the rest to me. My shortness of breath eased. She was very helpful and professional.

After I rinsed off, she handed me a warm, dry towel to use while she maneuvered herself into the shower to begin drying my legs off with another towel. Feeling warm and squeaky clean, I then walked over to the mirror and she began cleaning the dressings on my face. She washed my face the best she could, utilizing 2 x 2 gauze dressings and Q-tips to clean the areas close to the sutures. She asked me to hold on to the basin of the sink while she lathered up my hair with a shampoo that mysteriously required no water. She didn't rush through it like many nurses later did. She did a thorough and efficient job. She left me to comb my own hair, finally clean enough to lie right on my head for the first time in days.

"You are clean as a whistle now. I brought you a couple of fresh gowns so that you can change whenever you want. Do you need anything else?" she asked.

"I can't think of anything," I replied. "I really appreciate your help." I felt like a million bucks all of a sudden. I looked a hell of a lot better too.

*　　*　　*

After a couple of days in the hospital I started getting a lot of phone calls and even get-well cards and notes. Apparently some of the calls were going to my parents' home first. Some of my friends thought it might be better to check in with my mother to see how I was doing before calling me. When my friends called and asked how I was doing, I generally replied that I was doing fine. A few friends told me they were shocked at the energy level in my voice, because after speaking with my mother they were under the impression that I was not in the greatest shape and not really up to seeing people just yet. That was when I discovered that my mother was not only being protective of me and sensitive to the fact that I might not want to see just any friend who called, but it seemed that she might be afraid that should my friends come see me, their reactions might upset me. This thought made me feel embarrassed about myself. I began to consider that I must have looked pretty unsightly after all. For the first time, I was overwhelmed with uncertainty about how I really looked to other people. But my mother's comments agitated me as well.

Why couldn't she have let me tell my friends first how I really felt?

After a couple of these phone calls, I confronted my mother. "What gives you the right to decide for me who I want to see and who I don't want to see? I'm not gunna hide out and become a recluse because I'm afraid my friends won't be able to handle it. If someone wants to see me, let me make the decision. Don't decide for me."

Her reply was very apologetic. "I'm sorry honey. I was just trying to help. I'll give them your number for now on."

*   *   *

I was happy that I had friends that were willing to come see me. I knew that seeing me for the first time would be hard for them, but the last thing I wanted to do was discourage them. Friends and family were what made life worth living. And I certainly wasn't excited about sitting in bed all day and seeing only the same old faces. I loved my family, but seeing friends was important too.

I wasn't afraid to tell friends about my condition. I had been afraid before surgery. It had been difficult for me to tell people that I had been diagnosed with cancer and that I was going to have surgery. But now that the surgery was over and the margins were clean, I felt like telling and seeing everyone. The surgery had been successful. Sure, I looked like a monster, but I knew that was only temporary. In a few months I'd be back to Terry. I was sure. Reconstructive surgeons and plastic surgeons were able to do amazing things. That's what I had read and heard, anyway.

Before the surgery I felt like I had lost a battle. I had fought with cancer and it had gotten the best of me. I wasn't proud of that. I felt like something was wrong with me for getting cancer. It was my fault. It was something in my mind or the stress that I couldn't handle that caused it. It was a failure of mine, and I hated failure.

I was always competitive. I wanted to get good grades in school. I wanted to be a top performer in athletics. I had a lot of goals and aspirations. When I realized that I had a serious cancer that could possibly kill me, I felt like I had been cut from the team, or given an "F" by the teacher. It made me feel like a loser to have to tell people that I had cancer and would need major surgery and radiation treatment to cure it.

Now, all of a sudden, I felt refreshed, like I had beaten this evil being, finally. I was on top again. I wanted to talk to friends. I was sure the worst was behind me.

*   *   *

In the days that would follow, I started getting so many notes, cards and flowers, it was overwhelming. I was getting cards from distant relatives and even from people that I hadn't seen in years. Some weren't even friends anymore. Word was traveling fast. It made me wonder what people were really saying about me. But I was touched by it too, especially by the fact that the cards weren't being mailed to my home address in care of my mother or anything. People made the effort to get the cards off right away and directly to my hospital room. Perhaps word had spread that I was dying and people were saying 'you better get that card off right away, before he's gone.' Interestingly, I still hadn't heard a word from Kerri. I thought she would have been the first person to call or come see me.

The first night I saw anyone outside of my family was when John, Tyler and Rich showed up with their girlfriends. I was a little surprised that the girls had come along, but I knew them well. Fortunately, Jennifer and Allison were not the serious types. In fact, both had a great sense of humor.

When someone has a sense of humor, it makes his or her visit to the hospital so special. Laughing is such great therapy. My only concern after laughing so much at the beginning of their visit was that my sutures were going to pop out. I had actually asked my nurse the first day if laughing would cause any problems with my sutures. She'd said that laughing was okay, but if I had to sneeze, I should try like hell to prevent it.

Why was it okay to laugh but not sneeze? What was really that different about laughing and sneezing, at least as it related to my condition and the fact that I had sutures along my nose, cheek and upper lip? I determined that sneezing was more abrupt and forceful and would create pressure on the facial muscles and nose. But I also knew that I had had many a laugh that distorted just about every muscle in my face. I decided that the reason laughing was okay was because a good laugh every day was always recommended as good therapy and therefore it could never be a bad thing.

When my friends arrived that night, I had just been given my dinner. On the tray sat a carton of fruit juice, a milk shake, warm tea, water, and an assortment of purees. The purees were whatever was on the regular dinner menu, i.e. carrot puree, Swiss steak puree and potatoes. The thought of eating anything but the potatoes made me sick to my stomach, especially the pureed steak. Ugh! I knew I should eat everything to get my strength back, but unless it had an acceptable consistency or tasted decent, I couldn't do it. I realized that I had the same food as everyone else, but when food was pureed it just didn't taste the same. It would be like eating warm, melted ice cream. No, thanks.

I tried to amuse my friends as much as they tried to amuse me. I had to show them that I could drink my grape juice through a straw and funnel it right back out my nose. Though not an attractive site to watch, I thought it was funny. I guess it was show and tell time for me. I also wanted them to see that I still had a sense of humor.

Because I had lost part of my hard palate, I had to be careful not to let the fluid or food under my obturator or it would work its way out my nostril, which wasn't really a nostril. My right nostril consisted of just a little air hole that opened up into my mouth. My other nostril also partially opened into my palate, and that was the reason that food and fluids could drain out through my "nostrils" whenever I ate or drank.

I was still on morphine and while my friends were there visiting with me I received another shot. They stayed about an hour and then noticed I was fading into the world of never-never land and so said their good-byes.

I didn't remember much of what we talked about in my room that night, but the next morning when I woke up I felt good. The prior night's visit had been my first with friends. It was comfortable even though I was a little insecure about my appearance. No one gloated over my dressings or my sutures or my flap. They acted as if I looked like the Terry they had known before.

I was a little nervous prior to their visit. If their jaws had dropped when they walked in or if they had acted uneasy at all in my room, I would have known right away that what had happened to me was more horrific than I had at first thought. I realized I wasn't that bad off, because I still had my friends and they had made me feel like I was still a whole person. Another milestone had been accomplished. I was going to be okay.

Reading the paper the next morning was a little more comprehensible than the days before. The anesthetic had worn off and I was getting used to the medication prescribed to me. I finally wanted to read again and the words, sentences and paragraphs were starting to make sense. I didn't feel like I was in a fog as much as before.

That afternoon I had another new nurse. Adrienne walked in to my room around 4:00 that day and introduced herself as the nurse that would be caring for me that evening. Adrienne was the innocent, somewhat shy type who needed just a little prodding to open herself up. Once she knew you though, she was very talkative and sensitive.

Adrienne was about twenty-six years old, and had a very childlike but cute smile, and beautiful, big brown eyes. She had a soft voice, and like all the nurses at UCSF, Adrienne seemed very committed to the patient's well being. Because UCSF was my first experience with nurses on a regular basis, I just figured that all nurses were as sensitive and personable as the ones caring for me. As I later discovered when I had surgery in other hospitals, the nursing staffs fell far short of UCSF's standards.

At other hospitals that I would later receive care from, I found it difficult to get what I needed. Usually, the nursing staffs wouldn't even check on me periodically like they did at UCSF. They checked on me as the schedule required, but if I needed something, I had to beep them. Oftentimes, beeping them once wasn't even enough. I would beep over and over again for help before someone would come in, and when finally someone would respond, it would be with an irritated look and tone of voice. The response would generally be a negative one—"What's the problem?"—rather than "How can I help?" There were exceptions to this, but it was hard for anyone to measure up to the caregivers at UCSF.

Good hospital care (professionalism, good medicine and sensitivity to the patient) plays a huge part in a patient's recovery and outlook. The experience at UCSF was not a dreadful one like many might expect. In certain hospitals I believe it could be dreadful. At UCSF my attitude was affected by the attitudes of those caring for me. I strongly believe that recovery and healing and getting well are impacted by the people around you and the energy and spirit they bring with them. If that energy is positive it will enhance your own spirit and well being.

I received a lot of positive energy that night in the hospital from Adrienne. She kept telling me that I had a great attitude and that I was strong, mentally and physically. We talked about religion a little bit and I told her that my faith in God was something that was helping me get through this ordeal.

The next night Adrienne was my nurse again, and she remembered our conversation about faith and prayer. At about 10:00 p.m., as the lights generally go out and the patients are encouraged to go to sleep for the night, Adrienne made her final visit to my room. She cleaned my dressings, checked my vitals and then walked to the door and closed herself into my room. The lights were out. She returned to my bedside and pulled a chair next to my bed.

Adrienne must have known I would be open to what she was about to do. She grabbed my hands and cupped them in hers and told me she wanted to say a little prayer with me. As she spoke, I closed my eyes and listened to her soft voice. She prayed for my health and strength and prayed for courage to get me back on my feet and back to my life. We prayed together for about ten minutes.

Adrienne then stood up, and with a nice smile said, "Sleep well. Have nice dreams. I'll check on you in a couple hours."

I thanked Adrienne for her prayers and for the time she spent with me. I was so relaxed, I immediately fell off to sleep, something I had not been able to do in the hospital until that night. It usually took me about forty-five minutes before I could doze off. I was blessed to have Adrienne as a nurse.

*   *   *

I had been given the green light to walk as much as I desired, so I started walking after breakfast, lunch and dinner, as well as a few times in between. Only a week prior, I had been running four days a week, playing three-on-three basketball and lifting weights regularly. I wasn't going to let all that hard work go down the drain. Walking wasn't as much fun or as good of exercise as those other things, but I was determined to do what I could to get myself back to Terry as soon as I could.

My walks represented an interesting study. I began to understand again that there was another world outside of my hospital room. Though it wasn't the real world, I realized it was a stepping stone to it. I wanted to walk, the nurses encouraged me to walk, but the other patients and guests in the hallways oftentimes gave me looks that made me wonder if I should be hiding out in my room instead. My friends and family hadn't given me those looks of shock and amazement that I received from other people.

I walked circuits around Fourteen Long (the 14th floor of Long Hospital at UCSF). (Moffitt and Long Hospitals both reside at UCSF). I would walk the same routes, either clockwise or counterclockwise. Fortunately, the floor I was on was a pretty big wing of the hospital dedicated just to patient rooms. Therefore, the hallways were long and you didn't have to cross into another care area unless you walked a great distance.

As I walked, I had to use my left eye for direction, as my head was tilted down and to the right. I would see people coming towards me and sometimes they would jump out of my way and their jaws would drop open, as if in shock. I was embarrassed, but I kept reminding myself that it was only temporary. Dr. Cravens had told me he'd reconstruct me back to the "real" Terry. I had to just ignore the looks. It was only temporary.

I was off the morphine and it was really a great relief. Though it was very relaxing, and an enjoyable high, I had some strange experiences that I knew were related to the drug.

Two nights in a row I woke up in deep sweats and out of breath. Both nights I dreamt almost the same thing. I was a spider climbing up the wall in my hospital room. As I climbed up onto the ceiling, I was able to turn over and continue to walk myself on all fours until I was exactly over my bed. I watched myself lying in the hospital bed asleep. In the dream, I started to panic as I began to realize I had left my body. Was I dead? Oh, shit! I had seen this kind of stuff on television. Wasn't this type of experience a somewhat common one for people who die on operating tables briefly and then come back to life? These were the thoughts going through my head in the dream.

When I awoke, I was able to calm down, but only after I started wondering why I would have that kind of dream. Was this a signal that I was going to die? I shrugged it off the first night and went back to sleep.

The next morning I had to tell my brothers about the dream.

But as I recounted the dream to them I described it more as a cool drug trip rather than a frightening wake up call that maybe my days were numbered.

The next night I had almost the exact same dream. When I woke up sweating and out of breath again, I wondered if this was going to become a recurring nightmare or if it meant God was telling me something and preparing me for my final days. As I collected myself, I realized that these thoughts in my head were ridiculous. The doctor told me everything looked good and he was pretty sure he had gotten everything. 'These were just dreams,' I told myself, 'and dreams don't have to mean anything.'

The next morning after breakfast and my walk I took a nap. At the foot of my bed hung a grouping of balloons—balloons with designs and words on them, like smiling faces and "get well" wishes. Once again, I had a dream that scared me to death.

As I fell asleep and began dreaming, the red and purple balloons turned into bloody red and evil faces of the devil. As I lied in my bed looking out into the blackness of night, five or six faces of the devil appeared and started bobbing back and forth at me, laughing at my sorry state. I woke up again sweating and panting.

'Why these horrible nightmares?' I asked myself. Rarely in my life did I have nightmares. As a child I remembered having a few, but they were few and far between. I had had three in two days and that afternoon I was destined for another.

I seemed to be very tired that particular day and I was beginning to wonder if I really needed the morphine anymore. I knew it made me sleepy, and I was getting tired of sleeping during the day. I was ready to be normal again. I was willing to deal with a little pain. If it really hurt I could always go back to it. But why not try to wean myself off of it? The nurses and doctors sure weren't trying to take it away from me. But why?

As I fell asleep again that afternoon, I had the most memorable nightmare of all. Everything was purple. Somehow I had left my hospital room to run an errand for myself. I had only a purple hospital gown on and I was carrying my IV stand as the purple, grape-juice-like IV solution dripped into my arm. As I was outside of the building on my way to wherever it was I was going, I suddenly realized I was completely lost. I had no idea what city or town I was in and there was no one for me to ask. It was getting dark and it was beginning to snow. I was going to freeze to death. I was hopelessly alone, my medication was running low and I thought I was going to die. It was as if a nuclear bomb had dropped. There were no people anywhere and nothing I looked at was even remotely familiar. I could see myself in the dream. It was as if I was watching a video of myself.

For the first time in a dream, I saw myself as the 'new' Terry. I had the same disfigurement in the dream as I did in real life. The flap hung from my face down to my shoulder as I strode up and down streets, looking to find my way to wherever it was I was going. But when I realized I didn't know where I was going, that my destination no longer was clear, I decided that I had to get back to the hospital. I was going to get an infection. Why did I leave my room? What the hell was I trying to find in this desolate town? Perhaps I was trying to get away from everything. Maybe I was just trying to find a place to hide.

Was I trying to escape from the mess I was in? Was the dream telling me I couldn't, or I shouldn't? I was lost and I needed to return to the real world. Escaping was not the answer. I felt like I was hallucinating.

I called for my nurse and Adrienne came into my room right away.

"I am having these horrible dreams and all I can think is that the morphine is doing it to me. Can you put a note in my file that I have requested no more morphine?"

"I will check with your doctor, but I think if you feel you don't need it now, you'll probably be okay. Just let me know if you feel any pain at all. There are other pain killers we can give to you that might be easier on you."

*　　*　　*

Because most of my friends were still into going to school or work and then going out for a few drinks in the evenings, they were working their visits to the hospital around spending the night on the town or at least visiting bars close to UCSF that normally they wouldn't go to—places like Edinburgh Castle and Pat O'Shea's on Geary Street. It worked out perfectly really. Friends would come by around 6:00 or 7:00, stay until 8:30 or so and then head out in prime time to hit the bars.

That is not to say that friends wouldn't come by unless they had other plans, but at least it didn't make me feel guilty that they were heading all the way into the far part of the city just to see me. But guys like Sam Hooker and Liam and Tom and my brother Rob would oftentimes show up in the middle of the day with a milk shake for me and that was a real treat. Milk shakes were about the only things I could have that tasted good and went down easy. I was losing weight, so there was definitely no guilt in wolfing down high fat milk shakes. But I think they realized that seeing me during the day would be a nice surprise for me given that my days laying in bed were sometimes very long and boring. It really meant a lot to me to see friends who would use up their lunch hours to fight traffic over to UCSF just to say hi. Still, I hadn't heard from Kerri.

That next night there were a few guys coming over to see me. Rob had told Jim and Mike to stop by after 6:30 that night so that I would be finished with dinner and able to visit with them easier. Unfortunately, the doctor had stopped by right around 5:30 to check on me (which was when my floor served dinner to patients), and before I knew it, my dinner had been sitting on my tray for forty-five minutes and it was already nearing 6:30. I tried to eat the purees, but I was still having trouble getting food down and the process of eating a meal could still take me an hour. So, not only did the food taste bad, but it was cold. I guess that was another reason I liked milk shakes so much—they were already cold, and I somehow found a way to get those down before they ever got warm.

Sure enough, just as I started eating, Jim and Mike showed up with Rob. When Rob, Jim and Mike got going on different subjects, you needed a power outage to stop them. They would start play-acting and the laughing would start and never let up. Between laughing and trying to eat my dinner, Rob quickly realized that the latter wasn't happening. I couldn't eat and laugh at the same time.

Rob put his hands up and motioned to Jim and Mike. "All right, guys. Let's let Terry eat his dinner. He needs the nourishment. Terry, we're going to the visiting room down the hall for half an hour and then we'll come back."

After I finished dinner, I was able to spend some time with Jim and Mike. Both of them were very sincere and had very sensitive sides to them. The funny stuff stopped after awhile and we started talking about my procedure and what lied ahead for me. They were encouraging and positive. Mike compared me to other guys in the fraternity, saying that a lot of guys wouldn't have had the strength or courage to go through what I was dealing with.

I thanked Mike and told him I appreciated what he said, but told him my reaction to this whole thing was really just the natural human response. How else would I deal with it, but to deal with it? I felt strongly about what I was saying, but I also didn't feel that criticizing others would make me feel any better, nor was it the right thing to do. I knew now, for the first time in my life, that I might be the one criticized by people for the way I looked and I didn't like the prospects of that any more than being the one criticizing, which I knew I had done in my life plenty.

* * *

Early the next morning, Dr. Cravens strolled in with his entourage of residents. I started to wonder if Dr. Cravens had any life of his own. He was at the hospital late at night, early in the morning and generally on the weekends. He was obviously very committed and never seemed tired or irritable. His attitude was always very upbeat and positive. That attitude always managed to rub off on me too. When he showed up at 7:00 a.m. smiling and calling me "tough guy", it was hard not to smile and realize that life wasn't all that bad. He had a way of waking me up and still not finding me on the wrong side of the bed. He really didn't give me a chance to say, "Oh, doctor. I feel like shit." That wouldn't have been acceptable. And if he had a way of making me feel good in the morning, maybe there was a reason to feel good.

Would he have been that upbeat with me if my condition and prognosis were poor? I didn't know, but regardless, his attitude always made me feel like I was doing pretty well. If my doctor didn't smile or wasn't upbeat, I would probably be depressed or concerned about my prospects. Good or bad, his attitude helped me mentally and emotionally, and I know that in turn helped me physically.

It had been a week since the surgery and Dr. Cravens wanted to start testing my flap to see if it was close to developing its own blood supply. He told me he was going to tie a string tightly around the flap, about halfway between my nose and my chest. He could tell by the color of the flap after a couple of minutes if the portion attached to my nose had developed its own blood supply.

"Not quite," Dr. Cravens said after hitting a button on his watch. "It's turning a bit blue yet. As I indicated to you the day after your surgery, it will probably be a full two weeks from the first procedure before we can take you back into the operating room to cut that flap off. Besides, it gives pathology a chance to be sure they have tested all your tissue for any signs of remaining malignancy."

The bit about the tissue turning blue hadn't really even fazed me, but his point about pathology testing my tissue sent my heart racing.

"What do you mean, doctor? They're still testing my tissue? I thought my margins were clean."

"Well, Terry, I feel pretty good about it. But we want to be sure everything is examined thoroughly. It still could be a couple more days. But I wouldn't be too concerned about it. Things looked pretty good when we finished up the last procedure." He always put a positive spin on things.

I knew he was in a rush, and that was all I would get out of him about the pathology. So I asked about my "blue" flap.

"Is everything okay with my flap?"

"Absolutely," the doctor responded. "By tightening the string around it, I cut off the blood supply from your chest. By it turning blue, I can tell we need more time before the blood vessels in your nasal area develop enough of their own blood supply to support this flap by itself. Remember, this is a full thickness skin graft. Three layers of skin are being grafted, so it is a lot more complex than the single thickness skin graph we took from your leg and placed on your shoulder."

I shook my head to indicate that I understood.

"Terry, I also wanted to ask you if you wouldn't mind coming to our head and neck conference today? It is right across the street and we'll just have someone wheel you over there. Basically, I would like to show you off to all these other doctors and research guys. You'd be my show and tell. I think they'll find your case very interesting, since it is so rare. The reconstructive aspects of it are part of what I'd like to talk to them about today."

"Sure, doctor. I can't think of any scheduling conflicts today," I laughed.

"Great! I will let the nurse's station know the exact time, but I think we'll want you there about 10:30, okay? Hang in there buddy."

As he left, I felt a sinking feeling, suddenly being unsure of whether I would ever get out of this hospital. Maybe there still were some cancerous cells. If so, what was next? And why did I have to have such a rare form of cancer that I was the subject for today? Was I crazy to still be a happy person? Was I really just a guinea pig? What the hell was really going on? I began to wonder about everything all at once.

I was debating whether or not to tell my mother that the pathology testing still wasn't complete. What good would it be for her to hear about this stuff now? Maybe I would wait until the results were final. It would be too painful to see the worry in her eyes.

Mom arrived about 8:30 that morning and when I saw her I decided I would stick to the original plan and not tell her about my discussion with Dr. Cravens. She was breathing hard and carrying bags full of things for me. She was trying so hard to please me. How could I possibly drop a bomb on her now? She had a big smile on her face. She brought the daily newspaper, some new magazines and a strawberry smoothie—one of my favorite health drinks.

I did tell her about the conference. She asked if it would be okay for her to attend, and hoping I wouldn't upset her, I told her it probably would not be appropriate, but I assured her that it was probably not any big deal anyway. I really didn't want her to go for fear she would embarrass me. I would be in front of all of these intense doctor-types and I didn't want them to assume I was a little Mommy's boy who had to have Mommy by his side all of the time. I never thought to ask if it would be okay for her to join me. I wanted them to think I was strong enough to handle life's challenges on my own.

Kathleen was my nurse that day and she came in shortly after my mother arrived to say hello. Between the two of them there were more smiles in that room than white tiles. I began to realize that my mother was the greatest shot in the arm these nurses had. I don't think there were or are that many patients or visitors to hospitals that are as optimistic and upbeat as my mother. The nurses on that floor were popping in and out of my room constantly and I am sure it was primarily because these nurses needed therapy as much as the patients they were caring for. I would like to say that the nurses came to see me, but that would only have been wishful thinking.

I got the word that an orderly would come pick me up in a wheelchair to take me over to the conference around 10:30. Sure enough, a young guy walked in my room right on schedule and asked, "Are you ready sir?"

I replied to him that there was no time like the present. I started getting out of my bed, but he stopped me.

"Let me help you," he offered.

"I'm fine. I can walk over to the conference. I don't need a wheelchair," I replied.

"Sir, it is hospital policy to take you in a wheelchair. That's why your medical costs are so high," he laughed. "It's all about liability," he cynically informed me.

"Okay. Whatever you say. But I can get myself out of bed and into that wheelchair," I told him.

I situated myself, only clad in my hospital gown and ill-looking slippers that somehow had acquired bloodstains all over the toes on the right shoe. He asked me if I had a robe, as he planned to take me outside and across the street to the 400 Parnassus Medical Building. I got up and grabbed my robe, a thin-clothed and impractical Christian Dior robe that my mother had bought me. She thought it was so handsome on me. When I sat down, the orderly handed me two blankets to drape over my legs to warm them on the ride over.

The orderly knew the labyrinth of hallways through the hospital like the back of his hand. I could not believe how he was able to connect from one building to the next so easily without ever going outside. We went down the elevator one floor to cross a platform from one building to another. Then we went up the elevator to cross another platform. His goal was to get me from my hospital room to the conference room across the street without spending one second longer than was necessary out in the elements. When we finally reached a door to the outside world, we bee-lined across the street directly to the door of 400 Parnassus.

As he started wheeling me down the hallways from my room, he didn't waste any time starting conversation.

"What happened? Were you in a car accident?" he asked. That was the first time I had spoken with a stranger who didn't already know what had happened to me. Little was I to know that that question would prove to be the most common one I would hear from strangers who were just so curious they couldn't withhold asking the question.

"No," I answered. "I had surgery to remove a tumor." I struggled with my answer and I had to think why I responded the way I did so spontaneously. I hadn't rehearsed how I would respond to a question like that. My heart sunk when I realized that anyone looking at my face would now know something was terribly wrong with me. I was no longer the handsome, normal-looking Terry.

I wasn't ready to tell strangers I had cancer, maybe for fear that they might think I was doomed. Perhaps I just hadn't accepted it myself. By saying I had a tumor removed seemed less severe than to say I had "CANCER." I hoped strangers wouldn't ask the next question, which would be 'was it malignant or benign?' I hoped that the orderly wheeling me down the halls would be satisfied enough with my answer.

"Was it cancerous?" he asked.

I was suddenly getting irritable and I was barely down two hallways at Long Hospital. I was stuck with this guy for at least five more minutes. I was struggling with how I should answer the question. I didn't have a natural response, because I feared where the truth might lead. Everyone knew someone who had died of cancer. But this guy seemed like he might have been a pretty nice guy, if I gave him a chance to be. I decided that I shouldn't lie to him.

"Ya, it was." I realized two things from my answer. The first thing I realized was that I was going to have a hard time using the word cancer. I cringed when I heard the word. It hadn't bothered me so much initially when I was told I had cancer. But I guess now that I was facing possibly more surgery and beginning to understand how destructive and evil cancer was, the word truly frightened me. But the positive thing I realized from the answer I gave the orderly was that I spoke of my condition as past history. I could have answered, "Ya, it IS." But by reinforcing to myself that I was going to beat it and that the cancer was a thing of the past, I realized it was that attitude that would truly enable me to win the battle.

"Hey, man. You're alive. You'll come through okay." He had the right attitude too. But he also wasn't afraid to ask questions.

"Where was the cancer, man? You got dressings everywhere." He was seeing my flap, my shoulder dressing, and he had glimpsed the dressing on my leg that was protecting the single thickness skin graft donor site, not to mention the sutures on my face.

He was curious as hell, so I described in detail the whole ordeal, from beginning to end.

"That's major stuff, man. But let me tell you. You got a good attitude. You'll do all right," he said encouragingly.

When we reached the conference room at 400 Parnassus, he wished me well. I knew he was being sincere. He knocked on the door to the conference room and pushed the door open. "I have Dr. Cravens's patient here. Where would you like me to take him?"

Dr. Cravens hurried over to greet me and thanked me for coming. "I can take him from here," he said. "Thank you for your assistance." I noticed that Dr. Cravens seemed to treat everyone with respect, an honorable trait that many professional people lack.

Dr. Cravens rolled me up to the front of the room, which was a theater style meeting room. He began to tell the audience about the history of my medical condition and then began to describe how he was planning to use the extra tissue from the full-thickness skin graft to reconstruct my nose and make it symmetrical again. He seemed very proud of what he had done. He then welcomed everyone up to the front to get a closer look at me.

So there I sat, as one doctor after another looked me over and touched and pressed my flap. A few said hello, but mostly they just looked and stepped aside so the next person in line could see me.

As the meeting broke up, Dr. Cravens stepped out of the room to make arrangements for an orderly to take me back to my room. I felt much better after this meeting, knowing that Dr. Cravens was encouraged by the prospects for my reconstruction. It seemed unlikely that he would talk in front of his colleagues so optimistically if he had any doubts about reconstructing me back to where I was.

*　　*　　*

Because I had registered in the hospital as a Roman Catholic, volunteers often visited me from the Church offering me Holy Communion. I never hesitated to receive the host. I felt that Holy Communion could give me the strength and the courage to get through tough times. I liked to visualize that the Body of Christ would be digested and the life-giving molecules of the host would be carried by the bloodstream to all parts of my body to protect, to heal and to cure. Since I had been diagnosed, I went through this visualization process every time I received the host and it seemed to boost my spirit and give me more strength, so there was no reason not to keep up the practice.

About 3:00 that afternoon, a man knocked on my door and asked if he could come in to say a prayer with me. Before he entered, he told us he was a volunteer at the parish down the street.

"Come on in," I said.

As the man entered the room, our eyes locked. He appeared

to have a caring and giving look about him. His most striking characteristic was that he actually looked like the pictures we see of Jesus Christ. His hair, beard and features looked so much like how I envisioned Jesus Christ, it was uncanny.

As he approached my bed, he introduced himself to Rob, my Mom and I, and asked that we all join hands. He never asked what I was being treated for. He began to rehearse the "Our Father" and we joined him in concert. When we finished, he opened his eyes and gazed into mine. He squeezed my hand tightly and shouted "Take it away! Take it away! Take it away!" He paused. "May God be with you." He smiled and said good-bye.

We were silent when he left. I had never felt so much positive energy from one person in my life. I think my mother was shocked by his loud tone, but I thought his passion was what made all the difference.

I looked at my mother and at Rob and said, "That guy was intense. I felt his power." Normally I tended to be suspicious of people and wary of their motives. But this was an exception. I was on cloud nine the rest of the afternoon and evening. I really felt like this guy had some connection to God and that God was really hearing his request. As I lay in bed that night after turning off the lights, I thanked God for people like the "Take it away" guy, as I would begin referring to him as.

The next morning when I awoke around 7:00 a.m., I felt pretty good, but was beginning to wonder if Dr. Cravens would tell me about the pathology results that were still pending further analysis.

Not more than five minutes later, Dr. Cravens appeared in my room to check on me.

"How are we this morning, sport?" he asked with a big smile.

"Not bad. I'm feeling better every day." I responded. I didn't even want to ask him if he had the results. He would tell me when he did. Though he was always upbeat and positive, he was also a straight shooter, and didn't beat around the bush when he had to tell me something negative.

Dr. Cravens checked my various wounds, and even applied some Bacitracin ointment to my ears and nose with Q-tips. My left ear was beginning to get sore, but it was really the only sore spot I had at that time. Cartilage had been removed from my ear and grafted in my nose. Dr. Cravens said he had needed some cartilage to reconstruct what would have been my septum. It was encouraging to know that he had begun the reconstructive process because it was another signal that Dr. Cravens was confident he had eliminated the cancer cells.

He removed the dressing from my ear that had been there to cover the skin graft that had been transplanted to my ear from my groin area.

"You didn't leave much of me alone, did you doctor?" I kidded him. I had bandages in my groin area, on my thigh, on my left ear, all over my face, and all over my chest and right shoulder. It was no wonder someone would ask if I had been in a car accident.

"Actually, Terry, we still have a lot of cartilage left to use. The ears are made up of very useful cartilage for nasal reconstruction. Somewhere on those ears of yours there is a piece of cartilage that will match the ala that you lost. We can form a symmetrical nostril by using that cartilage."

"You are kidding. You mean to tell me that the right side of my nose will look just like the left side after the reconstruction?"

"Well, Terry, I would like to be able to say that. Sometimes it is difficult for the tissue to take if you have extensive radiation. I don't know exactly what radiology has in mind for you with that though—at least not at this point anyway."

After he left to go perform yet another surgery on some other newly diagnosed cancer patient, I suddenly began to feel like this doctor really was going to bring me back to the way I looked before. He was so confident in himself.

*   *   *

Around 9:00 a.m., after Rob, Mom and I walked the halls together, stopping to say hello to nurses and even patients that had become our acquaintances, I returned to my room for another day of reading and television.

Moments after I returned to my bed, a short man stopped outside of my room and peered in at me. He was also a patient, wearing his robe and slippers.

"Can I come in?" he asked my mother.

"Sure can," my mother replied. "How are you feeling today?"

"I'm sore," he replied.

"You look like the picture of health," she said.

"I had surgery on my penis. I couldn't urinate."

Suddenly there was silence. What does one say?

The man strolled closer to my bed, looking me over. He cocked his head sideways a little and asked me, "Are you gunna die?"

"No, I'm not gunna die!" I replied angrily.

"What in heck happened to you?" he asked boldly.

"I HAD cancer," I said. This was one guy I would never have said "I have cancer" to.

"You're not gunna die?" he asked again.

I waved my arm at him and looked in the opposite direction. "Get out of my room, okay. I really don't want to talk to you any more."

My mother stood up. "He's very tired," she told him. "I don't think this is the place or time to talk about death. We don't need that here." She put her arm around his shoulder and showed him out of the room.

"I never want to see that guy in my room again. Mom, can you tell the nurses to keep him away? That guy is evil."

A lot of people associate cancer with death. That was something I was going to have to start dealing with. But why should I let somebody I don't even know get the better of me? I couldn't let that kind of behavior bother me, but it did. I had to learn how to just brush it off.

*   *   *

The next morning the residents made their rounds again, led by Dr. Gambel. Dr. Gambel was handsome and athletic and probably the type of guy who would have been successful at any occupation he chose, given his demeanor and charisma.

Dr. Gambel and his colleagues gave me a good looking over and pulled back various bandages to examine the state of my wounds. They seemed satisfied that the healing was going along just fine.

"I understand you're not taking any more morphine or Demerol," Dr. Gambel confirmed. "Are you feeling any discomfort or pain? You know, we want you to feel comfortable in here."

"No, I really don't want to take any more. I think I'm okay with the Percocet or Tylenol with codeine if anything flares up. But I'm really not even in need of that," I told the group.

"Well, then, I know you're a college guy who likes to enjoy a beer now and again. I am going to go ahead and prescribe beer with your lunch and dinner, if you choose to have one. You can also have a glass of wine with dinner."

"That sounds great! It has been awhile since I've had a beer," I said.

"Actually, a glass of wine is really good for you because it helps with digestion and it relaxes you. The same goes for beer. The ingredients are good for you, in moderation of course," he laughed.

"So, how does that sound, Terry? You can watch the World Series and sip a beer at the same time," Dr. Gambel motioned his hand upward, as if toasting me.

"I'm all over it," I saluted him.

Unlike many of Dr. Gambel's colleagues, this guy really had

a personality and seemed well-rounded. From what I could tell of the other residents, many of them seemed like social misfits. They didn't even attempt to socialize with me or laugh when I laughed. They seemed so focused just on medicine, it was scary. In contrast, many of the non-resident doctors I had been visited by seemed fairly well rounded, despite their workloads and the serious nature of their occupation.

I began to wonder if many of these social misfit-type residents would ever be capable of becoming good, personable medical doctors. Would some of them drop out or would they pursue more research-oriented occupations in medicine? Maybe they would turn out like Dr. Kernan and never have any bedside manner. I supposed they could still become good scientific doctors.

I began to wonder if I would have the same confidence I had only weeks ago, before going under the knife. I wondered what I would be like as a person if I were permanently disfigured. Would I have the same confidence? Could I become a successful businessperson? I felt that I was going down the right path before all this happened, but what lied ahead of me? I had just finished a term as President of one of the most popular fraternities on campus at a University that was well respected. I was striving for balance, but now I had cancer and suddenly I was somebody completely different.

As I began to think about where I might be in six months or six years, I realized that those kinds of thoughts weren't going to help me to deal with my present condition. I had to focus on today and build myself up one day at a time. Why worry about the future right now? I had the rest of my life to deal with that. If thoughts like that were going to depress me, what was the use in letting them circle around in my head? I picked up the newspaper and began reading the business section in search of the day's hottest companies.

A couple more days passed and I was feeling better and better. Except for the flap dangling from my face, I actually felt like living normally again. Unfortunately, as soon as I began to feel better, it was time to go under the knife again.

The blood supply was sufficient for the full thickness skin graft to thrive on its own, so surgery was scheduled for October 14, exactly two weeks from the last procedure. I was told it would be a four and a half-hour procedure. After my ten and a half-hour procedure only two weeks prior, anything less seemed like a piece of cake.

Being prepped for surgery when I was already a patient in the hospital unfortunately made me feel like I really was "sick". It made me wonder if I would ever get out of the hospital. There were so many patients on my floor that had become fixtures and I feared I might become one of them.

A sadness crept over me when I was told the nursing staff would prepare me for surgery from my room rather than from pre-op. I thought how different this was than driving into the hospital the day of surgery. When I drove into the hospital for surgery I didn't feel sick and I didn't look sick. But when I was already in the hospital and brought down to surgery, I didn't feel that great to begin with, I looked terrible, and everyone on the medical staff already knew everything about me. I was not a new patient. I was just "a patient".

*   *   *

About 6:30 a.m. Carolyn strolled into my room holding up a needle like the Statue of Liberty holds up the torch. "Good morning, Terry. Are you ready for your morning shot?" she asked with a big smile across her face.

"What choice do I have?" I responded. Actually, I was very excited in many ways about having this procedure. It would be a huge step forward for me. The flap would be gone and I would start to look like a normal person again. I hoped, anyway. More exciting for me was that I would be able to leave the hospital so that I could start living again.

"Okay. Roll onto your side for me and pull up your gown," Carolyn requested. I was hoping that she would pull hers up instead. I was a dreamer. I did as she asked and in a couple seconds the prick was sending a soothing stream of Valium through my body.

Shortly thereafter, I was rolled down to pre-op and many of the same faces were there to ready me for surgery. I was feeling very good by the time I got to the hubbub of pre-op. Within ten minutes they rolled me into the operating room. When the anesthesiologist asked me to count backwards from 100, I tried my best. I made it to 99.

The next thing I knew I was in the recovery room. Unfortunately, the recovery room was the opposite of pre-op. I felt like hell, despite all the painkillers they gave me.

I opened my eyes and began to look around. Everything was coming into focus. Suddenly, I remembered why I had had surgery. I was a new man! I could turn my head from side to side and I could even nod up and down. I had a sudden appreciation for the muscles in my neck that enabled me to move my head. Now all I had to concentrate on was keeping my right arm to my side. The nurses had warned me not to raise that arm at all. If I did, I could pop out one or many of the eighty-plus staples that were holding what was left of the original flap down on my chest.

Upon returning to my room, I was able to examine and acquaint myself with the many changes resulting from the surgery.

What was truly amazing was how much the tissue making up the flap had contracted while suspended from my nose and cheek. As a result, when the remaining tissue of the flap was brought back to its original site, there were tremendous gaps between where the old skin had been cut and where the remaining flap of skin had been placed. The only tissue utilized from the flap was about a 3" by 4" area that circled my right shoulder. The doctor had planned for this in the first surgery and that was why the single thickness skin graft had been removed from my right leg and sutured onto my shoulder to begin with. I hoped the rest of my chest area would look decent once it healed, but by looking at it the first day it appeared like a bear had clawed at my chest and left two deep grooves from my right shoulder to my sternum.

The separation of the tissue made the staples look very unstable. The staples were huge, stretching across what appeared to be a 1/2" distance in some places. In the cavities one could see red muscle tissue.

There was a fair amount of concern that this 10" scar that began about 1" above my right nipple and 2" toward my sternum might get infected because of the exposed muscle tissue. About 6" above that stretch of staples another 10" span was also being held together by staples. Unbeknownst to me, the gap between the old skin and the flap skin on the upper span was even wider and would end up taking several months to fill in with scar tissue. The reason for the lengthy healing process was that the scar line stretched right below the collarbone, an area surrounded by a very thin layer of skin, which heals slowly.

My chest was a bit of a shocker to look at. Everyone that walked through my door had no choice but to see it. The doctor wanted the area exposed and not enclosed by bandages or by a hospital gown. Having it open also made it easier for the nurses to eyeball it to monitor its coloration and to simplify their cleaning process. When my brother Rob first saw it I remember his mouth and eyes widening and all he said was "Whoa."

My face actually didn't look a whole lot different. Yes, the flap had been removed, but little reconstruction had been done with the portion of the flap that remained on my face. It almost appeared that silly putty had been kneaded into the affected area. The flap tissue had more of a yellowish tint to it while the rest of my face was more ruddy in nature. The flap had been used to replace half of my nose, part of my right cheek and my right upper lip. The upper lip and cheek now appeared to have bubbles of tissue replacing the affected areas. The doctor had done an exceptional job on the bridge of the nose itself and the area that forms the outer socket of the eye. He had smoothly placed replacement tissue into those areas and the scar line was already almost non-existent. Amazingly, I still lacked any bruises on my face, and didn't even have a black eye.

As I examined myself in the mirror, I had mixed feelings. I was happy with part of my nose, but horribly dissatisfied with other parts of my nose, cheek and upper lip. I didn't panic. I accepted it because the doctor had told me he would get me back to "Terry." He suggested that it would probably require a few reconstructive surgeries to get me there, but I would get there. "We're going to make you 'streetable,'" I remembered him telling me. "That way we can let you out of the hospital. Later, we'll start reconstruction on the nose, cheek and upper lip. Then you will be Terry again."

When I had heard 'streetable', I thought I would look like a tough guy with noticeable scars on his face, but not necessarily a disfigured guy. I thought of Tom Berenger in "Platoon" as a guy with a 'streetable' look. He had what appeared to be a large keloid scar across his cheek that was suppose to have been a result of a knife cut from battle in Vietnam.

The reality of being 'streetable' became my first real disappointment. In some ways the cancer diagnosis had been less discouraging. Though I was not aware at the time, I was in no way prepared for what lay ahead of me. Had I known I would have been disappointed many more times, I may have had a less positive attitude about life in general.

I tried to shrug it off and regain my composure. My focus had to be on getting well and I felt sure that successful reconstruction would follow. I was blessed by my ignorance. I had no concept of the difficulties I would face in reconstruction. Just as I didn't understand the severity of my cancer at that time, I also didn't comprehend the complexity of what lied ahead in my reconstruction.

Lacking the support of normal facial bony structure, missing the muscles that defined my expressions and later being exposed to 6000 rads of radiation all magnified the challenge of reconstruction beyond my imagination. But I was ignorant to all that at this point. Therefore, I was optimistic and confident in my prospects of becoming Terry again.

The day after surgery I felt good. After I sucked down my breakfast (I still was having problems chewing) I got a call from my friend Tyler. This was the first call I had received since the surgery, and because there was no one in my room, I quickly reached my left arm over my chest to grab the receiver, thinking that as long as I didn't use my right arm the staples would stay intact.

"Hello," I said.

"Hey, buddy. It's Tyler. How are you doing this morning?"

"Actually, I feel really good, thanks. The surgery went well."

"Good. I'm glad to hear it."

"Hey, Tyler. I gotta go. Sorry. I'll talk to you later "

I dropped the phone on the floor as I gazed in amazement at the stream of blood flowing down my chest and over my stomach. "Holy shit!" I said aloud.

"Terry! Terry! Are you okay?" I could hear Tyler screaming into the phone as it dangled from my side table.

My heart started pounding. It was the first time I had been truly frightened in the hospital. I knew why I was bleeding, but the discharge of blood was so heavy, I was starting to panic. By reaching for the phone, I had stretched the incisions in my chest. The flow of blood wasn't diminishing. I quickly reached over and hit the 'help' button. There was blood all over my sheets. I was getting breathless from the sight.

Since I wasn't the kind of patient that hit the 'help' button very often, I wasn't thought of by the nurses as 'the boy who cried wolf.' Two nurses rushed into my room to check on me.

Their mouths widened in shock, but both nurses quickly shifted into action. The first nurse went into my bathroom and returned with dampened 4 x 4 gauze pads. She slapped several on my chest and applied pressure from both hands over the source of the bleeding. The other nurse raced out of the room, telling me she needed to find the resident doctor. I became more frightened as I watched them rush into action.

"God, I cannot tell where it's coming from. But don't worry. We'll get it stopped," the nurse holding the gauze pads said.

A couple of minutes later, the other nurse and Dr. Gambel appeared. Dr. Gambel was smiling. My anxiety diminished. Dr. Gambel's smile alone had put me at ease.

"What do we got here?" he asked me as he slipped some gloves on.

"I don't know, but I'm bleeding to death," I said, much calmer now, and trying to be funny and prove my tough guy image at the same time.

Dr. Gambel began examining me at once, instructing the nurses to retrieve specific instruments and supplies, as if he was doing surgery in the operating room. While one nurse acted as the courier for Dr. Gambel, the other cleaned the blood from my chest. She quickly honed in on the source of the bleeding as Dr. Gambel peered closer at the wound.

"I think it's a broken blood vessel in your muscle tissue. Nothing to worry about, but I am going to try to cauterize it," he said.

The other nurse quickly returned with the corderizer as Dr. Gambel continued probing around the affected site, careful not to pull out any staples.

As the corderizer was heating up, he explained that he was going to try to stop the blood by singeing the blood vessel. "I don't know if you are familiar with this procedure, but doctors use these a lot to stop excessive nose bleeds, among other things."

"Ya. I do know. Both my brother and I had that done when we were kids. I used to get bloody noses all the time," I said.

"Did you?" he looked at me puzzled. "Did you tell Dr. Cravens that? It seems a little coincidental that you would have had a lot of nosebleeds *and* this tumor in your nostril."

"Ya. I did explain that to the doctor, but he didn't think there would have been any relation because of the type of tumor I *had*.

He told me he thought the type of tumor I had was too aggressive to sit dormant that long."

I stopped for a moment to think about that coincidence. Could I have had cancer when I was a little kid, and just never knew it? Did I have a tiny tumor that didn't *really* start growing until just recently? It *was* a strange coincidence. As I pondered those questions, I began to smell the scent of burning flesh as Dr. Gambel burrowed his way into the gap in my chest.

"Hey, I can still smell!" I said. Though the smell was horrid, it was the first time that I was aware of my sense of smell since the radical surgery.

"All right! He can smell," Dr. Gambel shouted out the door. He continued to probe with his corderizer, but the blood continued to flow.

"You know, Terry, I don't think I can get down there far enough with this thing to corderize it. But, I think if we just put a stack of 4 x 4's on top of the area and have you hold them tight for ten minutes or so, it will probably stop bleeding," Dr. Gambel continued.

The stream of blood appeared to be slowing, so I wasn't as alarmed. For a brief moment I had wondered if I were going to watch myself bleed to death. But the fear had passed.

Eventually the bleeding did stop, but the nurses had to keep coming in with fresh supplies of 4 x 4's for me. I think I single-handedly helped Johnson & Johnson earn another .02 cents a share for the quarter on that one day. Frightened by my screams, Tyler had phoned back and been told by the nurse's station that I was temporarily unavailable to talk, but that I would be okay.

*　　*　　*

I began to feel better and better and Dr. Cravens informed me I could go home within a couple of days.

"God, I am going to get out of here. I am going to make it," I said to myself.

You hear about so many people that go into the hospital with cancer and never get out. I guess the realization that I was going to get out of the hospital really put me in another frame of mind.

I remembered the guy I used to run against from a competing high school that was diagnosed with leukemia and died within one week. He was strong and confident in himself one day and one week later he was gone. Life was so fragile. I thought for a moment and told myself that I would always try to remember how fragile life really was. We never know when our time will be up.

I was really looking forward to being in my usual surroundings. Given that it was only mid-October, the weather was still fairly decent and I figured I would still be able to spend some time outside. In fact, even though I had been trapped in a hospital room at UCSF where the weather conditions are generally cold, foggy and windy, I had been fortunate enough to get a private room with a view of downtown San Francisco and part of the Golden Gate Bridge in the background. Generally speaking, there isn't a view from UCSF because of the fog, but my stay was blessed with clear, nice weather. Almost every day I was able to lie in my bed and thank God for the beautiful view I had of the thick trees in Golden Gate Park, the tall skyscrapers from the San Francisco skyline and the golden brown hills of Marin County.

*   *   *

In a couple of days, I would be miles from a hospital. I was feeling better and better about my condition and prospects. What I wasn't totally prepared for was the reactions I would receive from other people when they saw me. But was it really their reactions that were so upsetting to me or was it my sensitivity and insecurity that made me feel their reactions?

CHAPTER ELEVEN

The Re-entry Program

When it was finally time for me to get all my things and check out of the hospital, I realized I had accumulated a lot of stuff. The flowers could be left, but I had books and posters, cards and magazines, cassette tapes and board games, all of which seemed to have a special significance and memory attached to them.

I got my hugs from Carloyn, Kathleen and Adrienne during their last shifts. They all wanted me to stay in touch. If they only knew how much I really wanted to stay in touch with them, especially Carolyn, they probably would have been shocked. Before I got dressed, I went to the scale down the hall to weigh myself. I had lost thirteen pounds in fourteen days. I hadn't really noticed it until I put on my jeans for the first time that day to get ready for the real world again. I was 165 pounds when I stepped into the hospital and I was a measly 152 when I was ready to leave.

As I dressed myself, I realized that besides being sensitive about my face, I now suddenly realized I didn't feel very good about my body.

Standard hospital procedure required that I go downstairs in a wheelchair, so I didn't argue. I was wheeled down to the main waiting room at Moffitt Hospital and then I was allowed to get out of the chair. The main waiting room area was very busy and as I watched visitors coming and going through the main door I noticed it was overcast and windy outside. People were wearing sweaters, jackets and overcoats.

Rob decided he would walk with Mom to get the car and suggested I wait. He thought I should get picked up in the front so that I wouldn't be exposed to the cold air. They were babying me, but I didn't feel like arguing, so I agreed to wait.

I found myself a seat and put my backpack down. As I looked up it seemed that everyone was staring at me. I suddenly felt very uncomfortable. "Is this what it's going to be like?" I wondered. I felt like the elephant man.

As I turned my head I saw two kids staring at me wide-eyed, one of them pointing in my direction. It must have been shocking to look at me. People seemed taken aback when they glanced at me. One guy looked at me and his head popped backwards and then forward as he peered at me to get a closer look.

If I was 'streetable', I suddenly wasn't very interested. I guess I wanted to be 'acceptABLE' or 'presentABLE.' I wanted to be anything but 'streetable' at that moment. What made matters worse was that it seemed an eternity waiting for my mother and Rob to show up with the car.

I looked down for a while, but curiosity made me want to look up again. Maybe someone would glance at me with no expression and keep walking like they used to do when I was Terry. As I looked up, a heavy-set woman was staring at me, expressionless. I looked her in the eye and she kept staring. 'How rude!' I thought to myself.

Suddenly, I felt like confronting her by asking, "What in the hell are you staring at lady?" I wanted her to feel as bad as I felt at that very moment. But that wasn't my nature. Not then, anyway. I looked away. In the months ahead and after countless episodes like this, my anger forced me to change my approach to strangers who stared at me or asked me questions about my face.

Finally, the Honda appeared. I realized I was sweating, I had gotten so worked up. As I stood up and started walking out of the hospital, I tried to keep my head up and I told myself, 'Every day will be better. The swelling will subside and you'll look more and more like Terry every day. It cannot get worse than it is right now.'

As we drove out of the city and headed over the Bay Bridge toward Berkeley, I was reminded that I was still enrolled as a student. What the hell was I going to do? Did I really want to catch up right now and add that stress to my schedule? I was already weeks behind when I went to the hospital in the first place.

I decided I wasn't going to worry about it that day. I considered going to Berkeley the next day to check on my classes and workload. I was going to have to gear up to leave the house though, especially after the reactions I received in the lobby of Moffitt Hospital.

Mom's birthday was a week away. I hoped I could do something nice for her after all she had done for me. As I thought about what I could give her, I realized her gift was really to have me home. That would be all any mother would want. Nothing else would seem to matter when you had had an experience like the one we were having.

It was exciting to finally be home again. I had my room again, my bed, my bathroom and, best of all, my choice of food when and where I wanted it. I was hungry by the time we got home and Mom had already anticipated that. She must have gone to the grocery store the previous day and thought of all of the things I would want. I was overwhelmed when I opened the refrigerator, then the freezer and after that, the pantry.

There was a myriad of different, hearty soups. She had made lime Jell-O, vanilla pudding and in the freezer I found a quart of Dreyer's Jamocha Almond Fudge Ice Cream. There was milk, yogurt, bananas and orange juice so that I could create any type of shake or smoothie I wanted. Based on what I saw, I was sure I would gain my weight back quickly. Everything I saw to eat was highly caloric. I still had the choice of creating pureed meals—vegetables, meat, potatoes—but the thought made me want to vomit. Besides, I figured I had suffered enough. I decided that if I felt like eating pudding and ice cream, so be it. I knew I would find a way to get a balanced diet by making fruit shakes mixed with powders and/or by drinking lots of soups.

Rob asked what I felt like eating for lunch. He told me he would make it for me. He wanted me to relax. I did not argue.

I told him what sounded good to me. About ten minutes later he was calling me to the kitchen. One huge bowl of broccoli soup (full of butter and milk), a bowl of lime Jell-O and a giant Jamocha almond fudge and banana milk shake. I was in heaven. If I had room left over, I could have some vanilla pudding.

After wolfing down lunch, I was more stuffed than I had ever been in the hospital. I quickly realized how tired I was once my body started digesting. I brushed my teeth (to the extent I could) and went to my bedroom.

Getting ready for bed was quite an ordeal, because it was time for my incision cleansing, Bacitracin application and changing of gauze pads. By the time I cleaned the incision areas with hydrogen peroxide and then applied the Bacitracin with Q-tips, it took about fifteen minutes. I quickly realized I had to become more efficient at cleaning myself. I hoped my wounds would heal quickly because the sooner they healed the less time I would have to spend cleaning them. Little did I know at that point that I would still be performing the same cleaning ritual, at least on my chest, for three more months.

I slept like a rock. About three hours later I woke up to discover I was hungry again. My mother had always told me that was a good sign. She worried that if I lost my appetite I might be "really" sick.

*   *   *

I was feeling much better being home in my own surroundings. I was eating better, sleeping better, and I had more to do. I could go outside on walks and appreciate the fresh air every day.

I still was a bit sensitive about being around strangers. Besides my scars and sutures that were still visible (Dr. Cravens didn't like bandages) I had packing in my nose which was a darkened red color due to all the bleeding I had had. I couldn't wait to get that out. Breathing through my nose would be a nice treat. I hoped for an even greater sense of smell too.

I was regularly visiting UCSF. I had to see Dr. Cravens and Dr. Zaring fairly often so they could monitor my progress.

Dr. Zaring preferred to be called by his nickname, "Dr. Z". He was kind of a 60's hippie type—very cerebral, mellow and quite humorous. Every time I went to see Dr. Z, he either made me laugh or he got me talking about his favorite pastime—sports. I always felt good whenever I left his office. He took care of me, he didn't make me wait, and he reiterated how important it was that I try to enjoy life and not worry about what other people might be thinking. He would tell me to "go out and have a few beers with your buddies" or "go see a ball game." What he made me realize was that life was short and I should do whatever I felt like doing, regardless of whether it was really prudent or wise. He often had a smirk on his face and he would tell me, "You're gonna be fine. All this bullshit will be behind you before you know it."

*   *   *

A couple of days later I got the packing out of my nose and I got the green light from Dr. Z to brush all my teeth. I no longer had to worry about my toothbrush rubbing against the healing tissue in my mouth. I brushed and was reminded of one of life's simple pleasures—the feeling of clean teeth and a fresh mouth. I felt like a new man.

*   *   *

The next day, late in the afternoon, I was in the bathroom cleaning my wounds when the telephone rang.

"Hello," I said cheerily, feeling better than I had in a long time.

"Hi, Terry. This is Dr. Cravens here."

"Hi, Doctor. How are you?"

"I'm doing okay, Terry. Hey, I am going to need you to get in here again for another little procedure."

I had assumed that my margins were clean at that point. Once again, I realized my ignorance had been a blessing. I had not been worrying about pathology results, so I asked the doctor what procedure he was planning on performing.

"Terry, on the top of your palate it looks like we might have to shave off a little more tissue. There's probably a few malignant cells left up there and I would like to get those out of there as soon as we can."

My stomach tightened and I felt a lump forming in my throat. I tried to remain in control. "Are you sure that is the only spot? Has all the pathology been completed?"

"Yes, Terry. That appears to be the only spot we need to go back to. This is not extraordinary. I would like to do it on November 5th, first thing in the morning."

"Okay."

"I will have my assistant call you back with the details and pre-surgery stuff that you'll need to do."

"Okay. I will talk to you soon."

"Take care, Terry. I will see you in a couple of days."

I hung up the phone. Fortunately, I was upstairs and had picked up the phone in my parents' room. Rob and my mother were downstairs when the phone rang. I was starting to cry. I didn't want them to see me crying so I turned around and quickly ran into my parents' bathroom and closed the door. I knew they would be up momentarily to see who had called.

I started crying hysterically. Though it was only the third time I had cried during the whole experience, I shed more tears and cried louder on that occasion than any time before.

I was frightened, scared and terrified all at once. For the first time I truly thought that I might die of cancer. I began wondering if my doctor would ever find an end to my tumor. I knew he could only cut so far. My right eye and brain were so terrifyingly close to where the last incision had been made.

Was I just destined to keep going back for one procedure after another? I thought of my parents. How would they be able to deal with this? How would my brothers be able to deal with this? At least if I died there was an end in sight for me. But for my family there would be memories of the youngest son. My poor family. Tears were running down my cheeks and as I heard my mother's footsteps in search of me, I cried harder.

"Terry. Is everything okay?" She could hear me in the bathroom. "Who was on the phone, honey?"

"Give me some time to myself, please?" I pleaded with her. I knew I wouldn't have been able to talk to her at that moment without crying even harder.

I felt horrible. I knew that every minute my mother was in the dark the pain she was feeling was multiplying. But I had to collect myself. Looking at my mother and seeing her loving and caring expression would only exacerbate my sadness.

After about ten minutes of hard crying, I felt better. Crying was such a great release. I only wish I had been able to do it more often. I walked downstairs and sat in the family room. Rob and my mother walked in and asked if they could sit with me.

"Yes. Of course," I said. I told them what the doctor had called about, but assured them that it would be a very minor procedure and that the doctor was confident he could get it all.

They both responded positively.

Mom said, "We're gonna get rid of this thing, Terry. There was a lot in there and the doctor could only do so much the first two times."

Rob said, "I'm sure the doctor didn't want to cut out more than he had to the first couple of times. He doesn't want to cut away areas in your mouth or cheek that don't need to be cut away. Don't you worry, Terence. You're gonna be fine."

They both made it so much easier on me. If either one of them had cried or had reacted the way I had—with fear or anxiety—it would have made it that much tougher on me. Their positive energy came from heaven. I couldn't have asked for better people to be around me at that time.

*   *   *

Though it had been less than three weeks since my last surgery, I was once again required to have lab work done and chest x-rays the day before the surgery. So, the afternoon before surgery, Mom took me out to UCSF for the one-hour pre-surgery check-up and check-in.

It is no wonder medical costs are as high as they are when you consider all the people and all the processes that are involved every time one needs to be scheduled for small operative procedures in a hospital.

You have to check in with one person. That person sends you to an examining room. Someone else comes into the examining room to take a blood sample. That blood sample is sent to some other lab technician to test. That person has to fill out paperwork on the blood and get the information all the way back to the doctor. In the meantime, you are sent to another examining room. Another attendant helps you and sets you up with an x-ray technician. Several x-rays are taken. The film is produced. Somehow all that paperwork has to get routed back to the doctor. After the x-rays you are sent to another examining room, where another fresh sheet of wax paper is pulled over the examining table for you to sit on. You wait for the anesthesiologist who eventually makes an appearance. He asks for your medical history and for feedback on your prior reactions to anesthesia.

*   *   *

After burning most of the afternoon at UCSF, Mom and I headed home. Mom was adamant that I eat a good, healthy and well-balanced meal the night before surgery. She wanted me to be as strong as possible. As usual, I was scheduled for a 7:00 a.m. procedure, so that meant I had to be at UCSF by 6:00 a.m.. After eating a ton, I went off to bed fairly early.

Though I was going under a general anesthetic, I was being sent home after the procedure. "Outpatient" procedures were getting more and more common because of the tremendous savings that could be realized by health insurance companies.

Dr. Cravens said that he expected the procedure to take about an hour, given what he knew about the remaining malignancy.

When I woke up in the recovery room, the first question I asked when I was ready to talk was "How long was the procedure?"

If the procedure had indeed been an hour, my confidence in my doctor and in my prognosis would be restored. If the procedure had taken longer, I would be concerned that maybe the doctor didn't know as much about my tumor as he thought, or that maybe my tumor would turn out to be anything but predictable. That was my greatest fear.

"Your surgery was about an hour and a half," replied one of the recovery room nurses.

I was satisfied. Dr. Cravens had said "about" an hour and procedures always seemed to take a little longer than expected.

"Did everything go as expected?" I asked the nurse.

"Yes. Pathology will still be examining your tissue, but the initial frozen sections they tested after clearing the margins appeared benign."

"Whew!" I said excitedly. (Frozen sections are tissue samples that are quickly tested for malignancy and the results enable the surgeon to determine whether he can stop cutting or not).

Given the brevity of the procedure, I felt pretty good and spent very little time in the recovery room. I was able to get dressed and leave the hospital a short time later. As I sat in the wheelchair being rolled down the hallway, I immediately realized how lucky I was. I could have had cancer in my leg or in my spine or somewhere that would perhaps leave me in a wheelchair for life.

I still had the use of all of my limbs. I would be able to run again, ski again, play basketball again, and lift weights again—whatever I wanted to do. Yes, I now had a deformity that everyone would see no matter where I went, but I could go anywhere whenever I wanted and I could go without the help of anyone else. I was very fortunate in a lot of ways.

*　　*　　*

I was taken to the patient waiting room where Rob and my Mother were sitting. Mom and Rob both had big smiles on their faces as I was rolled toward them. I had a pretty good feeling that Dr. Cravens must have been out to talk with them or they wouldn't have been smiling so much.

"Hi pumpkin," Mom said.

"Hello Terence," Rob said.

"It sounds like everything went as the Doctor expected, honey," Mom said excitedly. "He checked in with us right before you went into recovery. He said he only carved a tiny little piece off of the roof of your mouth. Does it feel different?" she asked.

"Not really. It feels like my plate fits the same as before."

"Cravens said you can eat whatever you feel like eating, so that is good news. I didn't want to see you have to go backwards again, honey," Mom said.

"That's great!" I said. "But, am I going to get to talk to him?"

"Well, I think he was heading into another patient surgery, but he told Rob and me everything. It sounds like there is nothing to be concerned about. We'll go home and have a nice lunch, okay?" Mom was so positive and so upbeat, it was hard not to feel good when you were around her.

I was feeling well after the surgery. The plate protected the new incision and that enabled me to eat as I had been able to before. I was still eating soft foods like soft-boiled eggs, cottage cheese, ice cream and fruit shakes, but every day I tried something a little more challenging. I was starting to eat pasta with light sauces because I knew it would be easy to digest, even if I did swallow some of the noodles whole.

*   *   *

A few days later the call came in from Dr. Cravens. I ran to pick up the phone upstairs in my parents' room as I usually did when I thought I would need privacy.

"Hello Terry!" Dr. Cravens said after I said hello into the receiver.

"Hi, Dr. Cravens. What's going on?" I asked.

"Well, Terry, I have good news for you. There was no indication of any tumor cells in the tissue we removed. That gives us the certainty that there is not any lingering cells left. Better to cut a little too much than not enough, right partner?"

I was suddenly relieved, though I hadn't been aware that I was really stressing about the results until that moment. A warm feeling rushed through me.

"Thanks Dr. Cravens. That is the best news I have heard in a *long, long* time."

"Terry, you just relax for a few days, okay. I am going to transfer you to my assistant and she can set up a post-op visit early next week. That way I can just make sure everything is healing okay. I'll also take a look at your chest incisions. Then we need to get you over to the radiologist for an exam and pre-radiation preparation. I am going to have my assistant set that up for you on the same day you come here so that you don't have to make two trips."

"Why do I need radiation treatment if you're sure the margins are clean?" I asked anxiously.

"Well, Terry, as I told you before, we decided at the Tumor Board that it is good insurance to have the radiation. Yes, your margins are clean. From all the pathology results, it appears we have removed all the cancer cells. But, radiation treatment should insure that any possible cells that still exist, cells that we may not have found, would be eliminated. I think Dr. Palmero, who is the Chairman of Radiation Oncology, will probably want to give you a pretty heavy dose so that we're sure we lick this thing this time. Your type of tumor is best treated with surgery AND radiation. Dr. Palmero can tell you more than I can about the radiation when you see him, so bring that notepad of questions you always bring me, okay." He giggled, chiding me like he always did.

That warm feeling of relief in knowing that the malignancy was gone lasted about thirty seconds after I hung up the phone. As I stood and looked down at the phone the relief quickly turned to joy and elation.

"Yes! Yes!" I said aloud to myself. I started trotting across the room toward the hallway and the staircase. Rob and Mom were downstairs in the kitchen. It seemed that neither one of them was racing upstairs as they had done the last time Dr. Cravens called. Either out of fear or kindness, they chose to stay put this time, and not race upstairs. When I was ready to tell them the news, whatever that might be, they would be ready to listen.

Hearing my footsteps clattering down the stairs, they both must have known that I had good news about something.

"Pathology was negative. Cravens is pretty sure he got it all!" I said powerfully, but between breaths because of my quick descent down the stairs.

Mom jumped up and wrapped her arms around me. "I knew it. I knew we'd get rid of this thing, honey."

Rob stood back smiling and said, "Congrats, Terence! 'Never Surrender'" he said, referring to the song we had heard in the car that now seemed so long ago.

*　　*　　*

My follow-up with Dr. Cravens went well. He was very happy with my progress. He sensed that I was somewhat bothered by the outcome of the reconstruction on my nose. I had been under the impression that the flap of tissue on my nose, cheek and upper lip was swollen and that it would start to look more like the other side of my face as the swelling subsided. From what I could tell, the decrease in swelling had altered my appearance very little. Dr. Cravens knew that I had hoped for better results, but he assured me that with reconstruction, I would be 'Terry' again.

I still believed in him and in his optimistic viewpoint, but I was beginning to wonder how he could possibly do it all in three reconstructive procedures.

"Don't you worry Terry. One way or another we'll get you looking like you used to look. But I have to tell you. You need to have the radiation first. A couple of months after that is completed we can do some more surgery. But we cannot risk doing any more surgery before the radiation."

I was getting a little impatient. How was I going to go back to school and back to work looking the way I did? How long could I handle the stares and the questions? It would be several months before I would look any different. At that moment I realized that in less than one week I had been told my malignancy was gone but I was already getting depressed about my future.

I had to stay positive. Being positive got me through all the surgery. I should have been ecstatic. The tumor cells were gone. Being alive was the most important thing. Why should I care what other people thought? Unfortunately, the reality was that I did care what other people thought. That was what was depressing me. I was depressed because I didn't feel good about how I looked.

As we left Dr. Cravens's office to cross the street to the Radiation Oncology Department, the biting wind woke me up from my deep thought. There was nothing I could do about my face for several months, so why worry? I talked to myself a little. 'Enjoy the free time. Stay healthy. See friends that are supportive and do what you want to do.' I was reminding myself to take Dr. Zaring's advice.

Suddenly I was feeling much better as I walked into the Radiation Oncology Department to learn about the next phase of treatment. The sooner I got going with radiation the sooner I would be done with the whole process.

As we walked into the Radiation Oncology waiting room, I was shocked. The waiting room was huge and most of the seats were filled with patients. Clearly, there were many people fighting the same horrible disease. I was far from alone.

One of the unfortunate things about radiation treatment, I would later find out, was that waiting around for treatment was depressing – the hopeless stares and tired faces an all too common site. And going to treatment would turn out to be a daily chore for six weeks. Though the task of getting to treatment and getting home would turn out to be a time-consuming regiment in itself, the waiting for treatment was the toughest part. Though I was given a 3:45 p.m. daily treatment appointment, sometimes I would wait one to two hours to get in for my thirty-second dose of rays. Watching the lonely, bleak faces while waiting was disheartening, but I quickly learned that smiling seemed to be the best medicine for everyone in that waiting room.

Only a few minutes after I checked in, the nurse led us into an examining room. Moments later, Dr. Palmero opened the door. He appeared to be around fifty, but still had a thick head of hair. His thick glasses somehow gave him the look of a man you could trust. He looked honest.

"Hi," Dr. Palmero said with a friendly smile.

We all said our hello's.

"How are you getting along Terence, or is it Terry?"

"Call me, Terry. I am doing great Dr. Palmero."

"Good." Then he was all business after that. "I have seen Terry's chart," he said, looking at Mom, Rob and I. "It appears you had a serious fibrosarcoma. Dr. Cravens did an excellent job. I must say he is one of the best there is. The radiation treatment I plan to administer is really an insurance policy. You might be fine without it, but with your type of tumor, it makes sense to have the radiation to insure that any lingering cells are eliminated."

At least Dr. Cravens and Dr. Palmero were saying the same thing. That was very reassuring.

"Given the type of tumor you had, Terry, I can tell you that the success rate with surgery and radiation is about 80-90%."

We had never heard statistics from Dr. Cravens. Dr. Cravens didn't believe in giving odds. I thank God he didn't. Had I known when I was being treated that my odds of beating my type of cancer were 50/50, I might not have had the attitude I had. Dr. Cravens never said anything but, "We're going to beat this thing, Terry." I believed in him.

Mom jumped at Dr. Palmero' statement. "What do you mean 80-90% for his type of tumor?"

"I am classifying fibrosarcomas, which of course are very rare. I haven't seen many fibrosarcomas in the maxillary area like Terry's, but I can tell you that we have a very high success rate in treating fibrosarcomas when the surgeon successfully removes the tumor cells. I think you should be confident that we can cure Terry. 80-90% is a very good number."

Despite the fact that I was hearing statistics for the first time, the stats were pretty favorable. I knew I could win with an 80-90% success rate. I smiled. I was happy. I was not concerned about the 10-20% chance that I wouldn't beat the cancer. Whenever I competed at anything, I always finished in the top 10-20%, not the bottom 10-20%.

Dr. Palmero then examined me quickly. He checked my mouth, my throat and my chest. He wanted to be sure everything had healed properly and that my lungs were clear. Radiation couldn't begin until my wounds were completely healed. But why was he checking my lungs?

"I need to send you in for another chest x-ray, Terry. Why don't we get that done today? And then next time you're in we'll do measurements and tattoos to prepare you for the radiation. What I mean by measurements and tattoos is that we have to measure very carefully the area to be radiated. We will give you probably two or three tattoos to mark the area so that when you come in for treatment, the technologist can line up your radiation plate."

"Wait a second. First of all, why do I need another chest x-ray?" I asked. "I have had a lot of these recently."

"Well, Terry, we have to be sure that your lungs are clear of tumor. Fibrosarcomas have a tendency to go into the lungs if the cancer isn't caught early enough."

Dr. Cravens had told me that before, but he had always said there was nothing to worry about because he had been certain he had caught the tumor in the early stages. Dr. Palmero, on the other hand, tended to be more pragmatic. He wasn't going to say something to make me feel good. He was going to tell me the way it was, and that was all there was to it.

The way he talked about the 'tendency' of fibrosarcomas to go to the lungs had a way of making me feel very uncertain all of a sudden.

'Shit,' I thought to myself. 'What if it had already traveled to my lungs but it hadn't showed up in the last x-ray? That must be why he wanted another chest x-ray.' I couldn't dwell on it for too long though, because Dr. Palmero's time was short just like every other doctor.

"Can you tell me more about these tattoos? I don't want tattoos on my face. I already have enough marks and scars that will make people notice me in public. I don't need anything more." I kind of smiled at him, hoping he would understand that I was a person with feelings, and not just a number.

Dr. Palmero laughed back at me. "No, no. These tattoos are nothing like what you would imagine. They are simply blue-green dots, each as small as a pinhead, but they are applied like a tattoo so that we have a permanent mark to use every time you come in here. These markers insure that your radiation plate is fitted exactly each time so that we radiate the exact same area every time you come in for treatment. These marks are also critical for you because without them there could be a chance your right eye could get damaged."

"What are the possible side effects of this treatment?" I asked.

I knew already about the possibility I would lose my appetite and therefore lose weight. In fact, Dr. Zaring had already warned me that I should be prepared to lose fifteen pounds over the six weeks of treatments. I was told I would have to be very conscious about eating right and eating enough, despite the loss of appetite I might encounter.

"I think in your case you will experience fewer side effects than most patients because the radiation will not cross any vital organs. A lot of people have problems when the radiation has to pass through internal organs like the stomach or kidneys. In your case we really only need to be concerned about your eye and possibly your salivary glands. The radiation could close off the salivary gland on your right side, causing dry mouth. We will be able to measure the area around your eye very carefully and I do not anticipate any problems there. Other than that you might lose some hair on the back of your head, due to the radiation passing through your skull and out the other side. I wouldn't expect you'd lose more than a little bit of hair. The most common side effect will be a loss of appetite. I would encourage you to talk to our nutritionist to make sure you eat the right things so you don't lose too much weight." He looked down at his watch, signaling that he was running late.

He told me to check with the receptionist on the way out for my next appointment. He then told us to wait and a nurse would take me to x-ray.

I realized that I was going to have a lot of ups and downs in the months ahead. I was excited that Dr. Cravens had caught all the tumor cells in my head and face, but suddenly I had to worry about my lungs. I'd been thinking that I'd had a localized tumor, one that hadn't metastasized, but all of a sudden it certainly didn't sound like a localized tumor to me. If it got into my lungs, I could really be finished. I wondered what lay ahead for me on this challenging journey.

My appointment was scheduled for the afternoon before Thanksgiving, almost two weeks away. Maybe I would be able to eat some turkey, peas and mashed potatoes by then. God, that sounded good. I hadn't eaten a decent meal in six weeks. I thought about the stuffing and the gravy and the pumpkin pie. Suddenly I realized that most of the food I was thinking about was pretty soft. 'Why wouldn't I be able to eat it?' I asked myself. 'Hell, my radiation treatments will not have even started until the week after Thanksgiving, so I know I won't feel any worse than I do now.' I was planning on a hearty Thanksgiving dinner. I would worry about Christmas when I got to it.

*   *   *

Having missed so many classes and midterms, I decided to make my withdrawal from Cal official. I requested a medical leave for the fall semester and indicated I planned to re-enroll for the spring semester.

The next couple of weeks went pretty well. I was feeling better every day but was still unable to eat much. I was walking and reading a lot more. I finally found that I was able to concentrate when I read. Unfortunately, I had gotten into the habit of watching "Leave it to Beaver", "The Walton's" and "Divorce Court" every morning. I was hooked. I was embarrassed about my addiction.

Almost a week after my appointment at the Radiation Oncology Department I still hadn't heard if the chest x-ray was okay or not. I hated calling doctors asking for results. I wondered why they didn't just call to tell me one way or another, so I could have some peace of mind.

I called Radiation Oncology reception to find out if they had my results yet.

"Hello, Radiation Oncology. How may I help you?" the woman with the British accent answered.

"Hi. This is Terry Healey. I am a patient of Dr. Palmero and I would like to check on my x-ray results please," I said.

"What was your last name again?"

"Healey. H-E-A-L-E-Y. First name Terence," I responded.

"Okay. Hold on please." She put me on hold and a moment later picked up the phone again. "Mr. Healey, I cannot seem to find your file. Can we call you right back?"

"Sure."

"We will try to get back to you shortly, Mr. Healey," she said.

"Thank you. Goodbye," I said appreciatively.

"Goodbye," she said.

I knew that the results were ready. How long did it take to get a chest x-ray and examine it, unless of course something was wrong? Maybe the receptionist saw the bad news and was instructed to have a doctor call me back. I started biting my nails. So much for reading the rest of the afternoon. My ability to concentrate was gone.

In less than an hour the phone rang. I picked it up.

"Hello," I said.

"Hello. Is Terence Healey there, please?" the woman asked. This woman also had a British accent, but much sexier sounding.

"This is Terry," I said.

"Hello, Terry. This is Dr. Corria. I am the chief resident here in Radiation Oncology. I was calling to tell you that everything is clear. Your x-rays look great."

"Thank you!" I said, exhaling deeply.

She told me she would be overseeing my treatment and that we would talk about it in more detail at my next appointment.

"That sounds great," I responded. "Thank you for calling. I'll see you in a couple of weeks."

Things were good again. But the seesaw would continue.

*   *   *

When Thanksgiving arrived, I was pretty excited. I was looking forward to spending some time with my family and friends on
a more celebratory level. I had been seeing family and friends a
lot lately, as they were constantly coming to see me to check on
my health and to be sure my spirits were good. But Thanksgiving
would be different. On Thanksgiving we often started having cock-
tails at about 4:00 p.m. and friends would drop in for drinks
until after 7:00. By 7:30 we were full of peanuts, chips and other
hors d'oeuvres, but somehow we made plenty of room for the
turkey, mashed potatoes, stuffing, peas, Jell-O and pumpkin pie.

I was even more excited that I would be able to eat most of
everything except for the turkey, and I wasn't planning to give
up on the turkey without a fight. I was also planning to have a
couple of beers: ice-cold Beck's hopefully. My brother Brian,
who had religiously come to see me most weekday evenings at
the hospital after he was through with work, was a premium beer
fan at that time and he was very supportive of my enjoying a
good beer now that I was out of the hospital. Dad had decided to
take the day before Thanksgiving off, partly because he wanted
to participate in my treatment process, and also because he knew
my appointments that day were a big part of the preparation process for the radiation. Because he was working full-time, he rarely
had the opportunity to help. Thanksgiving week was generally a
light week at his insurance company, so he wasn't that busy anyway.

At about 12:15, Dad and I headed to UCSF's Radiation Oncology Department to get my plates made. It was Dad's first visit
to the Radiation Oncology Unit and I could tell it was a real
shocker for him. I had warned him that he would probably have
to sit in the waiting room with all the other patients for an hour or
two, and therefore he should bring plenty to read. That suited

him just fine. He rarely had enough time to read *The San Francisco Chronicle*, *The Contra Costa Times* (the local county paper) and *The Wall Street Journal*. I was sure he thought he would have the opportunity to catch up on the news and all the other magazines he liked to read like *National Geographic* and *Money Magazine*.

But when we walked into the waiting room I sensed that he was feeling uneasy. Perhaps his ability to concentrate would be difficult given the fact that there were many, many children, young adults and his own contemporaries sitting around waiting for their own treatment.

If ever the American Cancer Society wanted to appeal to everyone to deliver the message about the seriousness of cancer and the need for donations, all they had to do was take a picture of this or any other Radiation Oncology waiting room. It was mind-boggling, especially when you began to realize that radiation patients look and act like every other human being. Yes, some appear sick, but many are healthy-looking parents and children that we commingle with every day, but never recognize to be sick.

Dad and I sat down, and because my father was so aware of my sensitivity to people looking at me because of my deformity, he restrained himself from glancing around. He picked up his newspaper and began to read almost immediately. I could tell that his actions were not natural. The quickness in picking out a newspaper and reading the first article that caught his eye seemed staged. Had he picked up the newspaper and scanned the cover page to decide what he wanted to read first, I might have been more convinced that he really did want to jump into his reading.

I opened up the Robert Ludlum novel I'd brought along and began reading. Moments later the front desk called for my appointment. I asked if it would be okay for my father to join me. "Of course," the nurse smiled.

From my limited experience at the Radiation Oncology Clinic, it appeared the staff was very family-support oriented. With the exception of Dr. Palmero, all the other doctors and staff seemed less scientific and more counselor-like, unlike the other doctors at clinics I had been to before.

Moments after being seated in the examining room, Dr. Corria entered. My jaw dropped. Dr. Corria, the chief resident, was probably in her early thirties, about 5'10" tall, short, thick, wavy hair and curves in all the right places. She was very confident in herself and her sexy British accent made it difficult for me to concentrate on what she was saying. I tried to listen and stop my daydreaming. I quickly realized her confidence was not unwarranted. She was sharp and articulate and had anticipated many of my questions.

She informed us that in addition to the 6,000 rads of radiation that would be delivered to me every day but Saturday and Sunday over a six-week period, the treatment would conclude with a 48-hour hospitalization, where I would have iridium implants implanted into my obturator. The idea was that these iridium 'seeds' would deliver the final, fatal rays that would kill any cancer cells that might remain. I would not be able to have visitors during those 48 hours, as I would be considered a 'radioactive' patient. This method of treatment might pose some risk of burning and blistering my mouth, she said, but I should not be concerned about sterility. Nurses and doctors would be allowed in to see me and monitor my well being. Dr. Corria had addressed any and all of my questions as she spoke. Though 'implants' sounded a little shocking, neither my father nor I were prepared at that stage to ask more about them. Hell, that was six weeks away, and seemed like an eternity.

"So how long is all of this preparatioin going to take today? I was told we would only be here two hours."

"It will probably take a bit longer than that, and that's if everything goes as planned. Sometimes adjustments have to be made."

"I'm glad you have plenty to read," I told my father, laughing.

Dr. Corria then escorted me to another room where measurements would be made on my head and the tattoos applied. I couldn't help watching her bottom sway back and forth in front of me as she led me down the hallway.

*   *   *

After the technicians were finally finished with me, I was led back out to the waiting room. There was my father, all alone except for one or two people who were still waiting for their treatments. As I walked through the door, my father looked up from his *National Geographic*. It was 6:30 p.m.. We had been in the clinic for five and a half-hours. Dad was smiling, though, and I could tell that he wasn't upset by the wait. But five and a half-hours was still three and a half-hours longer than I was prepared for that day. I needed to learn patience. My patience was going to be tested much harder in the years to come.

*   *   *

My radiation treatments were scheduled to begin in early December. I was also planning to go back to work the Monday after Thanksgiving. The law firm had left my job open for me. My supervisor had told me when I took the leave of absence that there would always be a job for me at the firm. It was nice not to have to worry about getting a new job, especially in my condition.

Things were coming together. I was going back to work and I was planning to enroll for the spring semester at Cal. I was ready for the real world again. But, how would people at work react to me when they saw me? How could I sit on the BART train for forty-five minutes and have people sit and stare at me? Could I handle it? There was only one way to find out. I would have to try it.

CHAPTER TWELVE

Trying To Fit In Again

I had closed one chapter in my life and was about to start another. Even though I was about to begin radiation treatment, I had already convinced myself that the tumor cells were all gone.

I went to bed each night and visualized myself standing in a mountain stream, while a crystal clear, chilling mountain waterfall splashed across my face. As it flowed over me it cleansed me of any possible remaining tumor cells that may have been fighting for their lives in my face. The cool, fresh water rushed through my veins, muscles and bones and washed the unhealthy cells all the way through my body and out my toes. As I stood in a pool of water, the current kept refreshing the water I stood in. The unhealthy cells were carried down the river, dissolving in the power of the blessed water.

My visualizations were not only positive reinforcement for me, but they also helped to relax me. The mental process helped me to sleep at night and sometimes even brought on wonderful dreams about being in the wilderness. I couldn't wait to backpack again and submerge myself in that refreshing mountain water.

* * *

When I woke up on Thanksgiving morning, I felt totally revitalized. I was a new person. I was no longer going to sit around watching television. Life was too short. I had goals that I needed to achieve. I needed some purpose back in my life. I wanted to finish school and start a career. I was suddenly more motivated than ever before to get into the best physical shape I had ever been in before. I wanted to feel *and* look healthy again.

Though I couldn't enjoy the Thanksgiving hors d'oeuvres, I did get to crack a Beck's Beer. The Beck's went down smoothly. Brian saw that I was finished and hurried out to the kitchen to get me another. He had brought an assortment of premium ales. He returned with an Orangeboom. I was content.

Fortunately, I knew how to control myself. I stopped after the second beer. Two was enough. I knew better than to weaken myself when I was about to start both work and radiation treatment.

I managed to eat everything in sight for dinner. Though it took a while to get things down, I even found it in me to eat some turkey. I wasn't worried about missing out on anything, either. Steve, Brian and Rob had finished their second helping and were about to start on thirds. Mom had made enough food to feed an army. I had all the time in the world to enjoy my dinner. A month later, I was glad I'd tried to eat everything and that I'd enjoyed it, because Christmas would be a different story.

* * *

The law office knew I was coming in from 8:00 to 1:00 on Monday. Liz, my supervisor, had told me that I could leave whenever I felt like it. She didn't want me to overdo it. I was a little nervous as I left the house that morning, thinking about the stares I might encounter on the BART train to downtown San Francisco.

I had to wear a coat and tie to work every day. Wearing a coat and tie gave me a little more confidence in my appearance. I assumed that regardless of the way my face looked, people would still perceive me as clean-cut and professional. I wanted desperately to be viewed as someone who contributed to society, because my disfigurement made me feel like I was less than adequate. My greatest fear was that people would think of me as a bum with no hope. I feared that I might look like someone who couldn't afford to fix the defect I had been born with. At least if I had a suit on, it would look like whatever had happened to me was only temporary. I jumped on the BART train and played the same game I had accused my father of playing in the Radiation Oncology waiting room. I grabbed the first seat I could find. I was uneasy and nervous. I immediately hid myself in the newspaper without concern for what I might be reading. I didn't look ahead of me. I didn't look next to me. I didn't casually flip through the sections of the paper on my lap. No way! I grabbed the whole paper and unfolded it directly in front of my face and pretended to be immersed in a news story, as if I had begun reading it on the platform waiting for the train.

The ride to the office was uneventful, given my refusal to look beyond my newspaper. If someone wanted to ask me a question about myself, I certainly didn't give the impression I was open to it. I got off the BART train and walked to my office. As I approached the main elevators with twenty-five other people, all crowding to get through the first doors that opened, I started feeling nervous again.

'People either stare straight ahead in elevators or they stare at one another,' I thought to myself. I just wanted to get through the first day without any stares. If I could get through the first day, any stares I got later wouldn't be as meaningful. But the first day was test day.

As the elevator doors opened, I stepped back and let the others crowd into the elevator. I decided to wait for the next one, even though I was aware that I was prolonging my agony. I was praying that the next elevator would arrive before the next entourage of people showed up.

As I struggled with my fears about the elevator, I realized that my life had become a dichotomy. Before all the surgery I used to enjoy the looks I got in elevators, especially from women. Before all the surgery, life had been simple. Suddenly, my life had become more complicated and scary. My biggest fear had now become that same stare or look from a woman. But the stare or look meant something entirely different now. In the pre-surgery days it might have meant attraction, but today it meant shock and wonderment. I was afraid that no woman would ever again feel attraction when she looked at me.

I remembered Marilyn, my first college girlfriend. I'd met her at a fraternity party during my second semester at Cal. I'd been talking with about five other guys. Across the room was a group of about the same number of girls. One of the girls was looking right at me. She was gorgeous. Suddenly, I realized that I recognized her. She had gone to a school in my district and I knew of her because I'd seen her at track meets that we both had competed in. She'd been beautiful then and was even prettier now. I looked away for a moment and then returned my gaze. She was still staring at me. I was excited. Our eyes locked.

Marilyn had beautiful, big brown eyes and heavy eyebrows. Her thick, long dark hair hung to her shoulders. She was tall, about 5'7", with long slender legs. Still an avid runner, she ran for the Cal girls' track team and could beat me in the mile on any given day. With confidence and self-assurance, I approached her. We talked the rest of the night. I walked her home. We kissed for twenty minutes outside her door. I wanted to go inside badly, but I also didn't want to blow it with her. We had dated for the next three months. But the stares that led to something positive, like meeting Marilyn, were gone forever. I feared stares now, because I associated them with pain, not joy.

I took the next elevator. I got a couple of looks, but I couldn't classify them as stares. 'Hell, everyone looks at everyone. It doesn't have to mean something is wrong with me just because they are glancing at me,' I told myself.

As I entered the lobby of our office, Tina, the receptionist, jumped up to say hello. She welcomed me back to work. As I headed down the hallway to the right toward my workstation, I passed the kitchen.

"WELCOME BACK!" came the shouts from inside. Streamers hung from the walls and a big sign read "WELCOME BACK, TERRY!" Most of the staff and some of the attorneys (the ones who didn't bill 23.5 hours a day) had been waiting for my arrival. Coffeecakes and pastries were in abundance. No one looked at me in shock. They all smiled and either shook my hand or hugged me. I felt good. I was onto the next chapter of my life.

*   *   *

I felt that working in the city again would be good for me. A lot of my friends, guys and girls, worked in the financial district. That meant we could get together for lunch or meet after work for drinks. I realized I had to move forward and get back into the swing of things. I had been used to people coming to visit me on my turf where everything was comfortable. Going out to bars was a good way for me to integrate myself back into society.

Friday, I worked until 5:00 and met some friends at the Royal Exchange. Though I thought everyone was staring at me, nobody said a word, and more than likely people didn't even notice me.

As I sat in the bar, I thought about the radiation treatments that would start the following week. I was very lucky really. Many cancer patients had to undergo chemotherapy, a form of treatment with much more serious side effects. I would still be able to visit bars with a full head of hair, normal skin coloration, and an appetite (I hoped) for food and drink. Many cancer patients weren't so lucky. Chemotherapy generally made your hair fall out, your skin turn gray, and, oftentimes, caused your stomach to reject many types of food and drink. It could be very debilitating.

When the next Monday came around, I was fired up to start treatment. The sooner I started the sooner it would all be over and behind me. I arrived to work a little early. I had planned to work from eight to three each day after my first day, because I had to travel across the city to UCSF for my 3:45 p.m. appointment. I didn't get to pick my appointment time. That was the slot Radiation Oncology had for me. I didn't complain. It was nice, because when I left work, I was done for the day.

One of my responsibilities at work was to pick up the mail in the morning. Picking up the mail involved taking the old mailbags down to the basement where the postal service employees exchanged your empty bags for your new mailbags. Usually, I took the elevator down to the lobby and then picked up the separate basement elevator with very little wait. But that Monday was different. Apparently, the postal service downstairs was behind schedule and had stopped the elevators so that they could ready themselves for the onslaught of office workers hungry for their two days of mail. As a result, about ten people were lined up outside the basement elevator waiting to catch the ride downstairs. I recognized a few of the people from days past, before my surgery. Even though we all sort of knew each other, at least by looks, no one said much of anything while we waited. But the woman next to me in line kind of turned and looked at me. I pretended not to notice her.

"God, what in the hell happened to you?" she asked, loud enough so that everyone turned toward me to look.

The attitude in her tone of voice so irritated me that I couldn't control my emotions. "It's none of your business," I snapped.

She wasn't going to take no for an answer. "Wait a minute. The last time I saw you you looked fine. Did you get in a car accident or something?"

I was shocked that someone could ask such a question in front of so many strangers. I'd promised myself that I would never tell anyone, "I have cancer," but that it would be okay for me to say, "I *had* cancer." I realized this woman wasn't going to quit and I wanted to shut her up.

"I had cancer, okay," I said thinking that would end the conversation.

"Cancer? God, what kind of cancer? Did you have skin cancer or did you chew a lot of tobacco or something?"

I lost my remaining patience and began to get angry again. "I had cancer, okay? Isn't that good enough for you? I had a rare form of cancer that started in my palate. But it's gone. I'm cured, okay?"

"God, how horrible," she said, making me feel worse and worse by the second. To say that what I had was 'horrible' made me feel as if what I had was something you wouldn't wish on your own worst enemy. It made me feel as if what I had was the worst thing you could have. And because it was my face, my identity, it hurt that much more.

Fortunately, the elevator doors opened. I rushed for the door, trying to position myself as far away from the witch as possible. As I rode the elevator down, I began to realize that she had probably spoken to me the way she had because she was miserable. Maybe it made her feel better to know that someone else out there had more problems than she did. I felt bad for not being patient with her. I had to forgive this woman and try to forget. She was definitely not worth ruining my day for.

I returned to work and tried hard to forget about the experience. If I stayed busy, I knew it would be easier for me to move forward and stay positive. I couldn't dwell on negatives or bad experiences.

But when I got into the elevator to go out for lunch, I thought about her again. Witch woman wasn't a one of a kind. Chances were that there were many more people out in the world just like her. How often was I going to have to deal with them and respond to their questions?

I took a quick walk to the sandwich shop, enjoying the cool breeze at my face. It was a cool December day, but the sky was clear. As I gazed up at the blue sky, I realized that I seemed to appreciate natural beauty much more now than ever before. I guess what they say is true. You don't wake up to smell the roses usually until it is almost too late.

*   *   *

At 3:00 I headed out the door for my first radiation treatment. I jumped on the "N" Judah streetcar that took me directly to UCSF. Though it took almost ninety minutes to get home from UCSF, I found it to be a very productive time for me. I got more reading done and stayed more current on the news in the ensuing six weeks of radiation treatment than ever before. Mikhail Gorbachev had become the Soviet Premier and the era of "Glasnost" had begun in the Soviet Union.

I arrived at the Radiation Oncology Clinic, checked in, and took a seat. They called me in for my treatment right at 3:45. I was amazed that they were on schedule. I was going to be very happy if my appointments continued to be on time.

I recognized the two technicians who were supposed to administer my treatment. I had met them at my orientation. Both were young, probably in their late twenties. The woman had messy red hair and freckles that made her look a little like a tomboy. She always wore a nice smile but looked a little tired. The male technician was dark-complexioned, with thick dark-brown hair and glasses. They both greeted me cordially and then got down to business.

"This will only take a couple of minutes," the man said. "We just need you to lie down here. I'm going to remove your obturator because of the metal in it. Then we'll get you positioned. All you need to do is refrain from moving, okay?"

In a couple of minutes I was ready for the rays. They left the room, and I heard him say from behind the glass, "Don't move."

A second later, I heard a loud buzzing sound. The acrid smell of ozone surrounded me. I almost gagged from the smell, but a second later it was gone.

A few seconds later the technicians came back into the room, made a few adjustments, and repeated the exercise. All in all, there were three buzzes of radiation. The technicians removed the tape from my head and returned my obturator.

"That's it," said the redhead.

"That wasn't too bad," I said. I was too cool to admit feeling sick from the ozone and I decided that I would ask one of the doctors about it. "Thanks a lot," I said, and out the door I went.

At the front desk I stopped to check in to see if I needed any paperwork or anything. The receptionist glanced at my file and said, "The only thing new is that Dr. Palmero has recommended that each Friday a doctor see you just to check up on you and monitor how you're doing. Just come in at the same time and we'll make sure you get checked before or after your treatment."

"No problem," I said. "Thanks. See you tomorrow." I was out the door at 4:00 sharp. Not too bad. The treatment was a piece of cake. 'Hell, I can handle this', I thought to myself as I opened the door into the cool wind.

*   *   *

Radiation went fairly normally for the next couple of weeks, except that sometimes my 3:45 appointment became a 4:15, 5:15 or even 6:15 appointment. I didn't encounter any other problems or side effects those first couple of weeks. I got a lot of reading done, and the waiting episodes also gave me an opportunity to meet some of the other patients.

There was one guy whose name I could never remember who stood about 6'4" tall. He had a large green "X" tattooed on both sides of his head above each ear. He had a mohawk haircut, so the X's were very clear on his white skin. At first I figured he was some kind of neo-Nazi. He wore black jeans and black T-shirts.

He was also very pale and skinny. I couldn't tell if this was from the cancer, the treatment, or if that was just the way he was.

One day, as the two of us waited for our treatment and it got to be about four-thirty, he went over to the reception desk. I couldn't help but eavesdrop on them. "I'm going to have to go. I guess I'll see you tomorrow," he told the receptionist.

"Can you wait a little bit longer? I'm sure the technicians will be getting to you in just a little bit."

"Well, my bus pass is only good for a certain amount of time and I need to catch a bus in the next ten minutes," he said.

"Okay, I guess," the receptionist said. "But let me check with the technicians to see if they can squeeze you in in the next couple of minutes."

I stood up. Even though I was eavesdropping, I felt it was okay to interrupt. "How much do you need to get a new bus pass?" I asked him.

He gave me a blank stare. "A dollar."

"Well, I have a dollar. Take it. And you don't need to pay me back."

I realized that he probably wasn't working and had very little money.

"You need your treatment," I said, handing him the dollar bill. "If ever you need to stay here late for treatment and you need another dollar to get home, just ask me. I'm happy to help."

A huge smile came over his face. "Thanks a lot," he said. "That's really nice of you. No one else would do that for me."

He was so appreciative, yet so pessimistic all at the same time. I guess he hadn't experienced many nice people out there. I felt that he should have asked the Radiation Oncology department for the dollar. After all, the delay wasn't his fault.

He thanked me again and then sat down next to me. Suddenly, he was talking and smiling like I had never seen before. Then he told me about his cancer. He had an inoperable brain tumor and the radiation had killed all the hair on both sides of his head, giving him the mohawk.

"I would never have cut my hair that way," he told me. He hated the X's, but they were marks for the technicians.

When he was finally called in for his treatment, I realized that I'd been just as judgmental as anyone else had. I'd had him pegged as a neo-Nazi when in fact he was probably far, far from it. I had learned a lesson. Even though I had been disfigured, I suddenly realized that I was just as judgmental as the next guy was. And I felt that I could deal with my own situation better knowing what I now knew. I realized that people aren't necessarily mean or evil when they say or think negative things about someone else. Unfortunately people get classified into certain stereotypes just by the way they look, whether intentional or not. I realized that day that we should reserve judgment on everyone until we have the opportunity to speak to him or her and learn what kind of person they really are.

The second lesson I learned that day was that if I expected or hoped that others would be less judgmental, I would have to set the example. We create negative environments just by thinking certain things. I should have been able to accept the stares and the questions from others because it wasn't their fault for staring. But I should also battle it by offering to educate others somehow, some way. If I could have responded to those curious onlookers by finding a nice way to tell them what really happened to me and to show them that I was as normal inside as they were, then I would have achieved something. Maybe there was a reason this all happened to me. If I could just remember to count to five every time I had a negative encounter, maybe I'd be able to remember this lesson and act accordingly.

*   *   *

The following week, after my treatment, I decided to visit my old stomping grounds on Fourteen Long to say hello to my former nurses. I figured that at least one of them would be on duty. It was a little after four o'clock, so I knew the shift had just changed.

I got off the elevator and headed toward the nurse's station.

"Hi, Terry!"

"Hey, Terry. How's it going?"

The nurses and administrators made me feel so welcome.

"I'm feeling good, thanks," I replied. "How's everything here?"

"Oh, you know. It's not the same without you and your family," said the nurse in charge of administration. She had gotten to know my whole family so well.

I laughed. I wanted to see my nurses but was embarrassed because everyone else was being so nice. I felt like it was better to say hello to everyone and to no one in particular. As my good luck would have it, Carolyn strolled up to the nurse's station to grab a file. Thank God, I thought. Now I don't have to ask if she's here.

"Hey, Terry," she grinned, finally noticing me. "How are you doing?" A tint of purple reflected from her hair.

"Hi, Carolyn," I said, trying to make it seem as if seeing her hadn't been my main purpose for stopping in.

We talked for a little while and I told her that my treatments were every day at 3:45.

Carolyn, being the kind of person who would say anything in front of anybody, then asked me, "What are you doing Thursday night?"

"Nothing that I know of."

"Well, I get off at four on Thursday, and there's going to be a Christmas party across the street from, like, 3:30 to 5:30. Do you want to meet me up here when you're done with your treatment? Then maybe we can go get a drink after or something."

"That sounds great. Hopefully I'll get my treatment on time and can meet you up here at four," I said, trying to hide the fact that my heart was racing with excitement. I really liked Carolyn.

"Well, if you're delayed just meet me over at the student union building—second floor. They'll let you in. And it probably won't be that big a party, so you'll find me."

"Sounds like a plan. I know you have to get back to work, so I'll see you on Thursday." I said my good-byes to the rest of the crew and went on my way. Adrienne and Kathleen must have been off, but maybe I would see them at the party, I thought.

On Wednesday, my friend Tyler called me at work and said he wanted to take me out for a Christmas lunch. I accepted, of course, especially given the fact that I was eating fairly normally and I hadn't seen him in a while. He offered to come pick me up at work and take me to the Hyatt Union Square hotel. He tended to be oversensitive to my illness, and I was capable of walking, but rather than pushing back, I agreed he could pick me up at my office.

Figuring it would be a long lunch, I told my supervisor I needed to leave at one instead of three and would make up the hours if I needed to. She smiled, waving her hand in a gesture that told me to not worry about it. She had said I could come and go as I pleased, as long as I let her know where I stood with particular projects.

Tyler picked me up right at one and we drove uptown to the Stockton Street Garage. We walked up to the Hyatt Union Square and got seated right away. We each had a beer and ordered some club sandwiches. Then Tyler pulled out a little box and handed it to me.

"Merry Christmas, buddy," he said.

"Oh, thanks. You don't have to give me a gift." I felt guilty as hell that I had nothing for him. He had picked me up from work, he was taking me to lunch, and he was giving me a gift. I, on the other hand, was doing nothing for him.

The box held a Brooks Brothers red print tie. I thanked him as he finished the last of his beer.

We finished our sandwiches and discovered it was already 3:00. Tyler had a real job at an insurance company at that time, but asked if he could drive me to UCSF to see what it was I had to deal with every day. I think that he wanted to really understand what I was going through and to offer whatever support he could. I told him I could just as easily take the MUNI, but he insisted on taking me.

"What about work, Tyler? Don't you have to get back?" I asked.

"Don't worry. I'll work it out. I want to take you over there and now is as good a time as any," he said.

He paid the bill and excused himself to make a quick call to the office.

We left the restaurant with plenty of time to make it to UCSF, but Tyler had the habit of pressing the pedal to the metal wherever and whenever he drove. He had so many tickets that I think his license was one ticket away from suspension. I gave him a hard time about it, but my words did little to change his driving habits. I figured one of these days he would learn his lesson. I just hoped it wouldn't involve injuries to him or anyone else.

I told him that they wouldn't let him into the treatment room, but he seemed happy just waiting in the waiting room. It gave him a chance to see how 'real' cancer really was. He saw young people and old people, and I think it was a bit sobering for him, but he wanted to see it.

Unfortunately, my treatment was late that day. He kept checking in with his office from the pay phone. They finally called me in at 4:30, and a few minutes later I was finished. Tyler said he'd take me home because he wasn't planning on going back to the office.

'What a pal,' I thought to myself. He had basically given up his afternoon without my asking.

As we headed down Parnassus Street toward Stanyon Street in Tyler's black Volkswagen Jetta, we cranked up his stereo as loud as the speakers could stand. My seat belt was on, but I started thinking that I'd probably end up dying from a car accident, not cancer. Tyler was an insane driver. He was hauling down Parnassus and in his attempt to beat the oncoming traffic, he punched it as he turned left at the green light yield onto Stanyon. As he made the left turn, suddenly out of nowhere we saw a woman about a third of the way across the crosswalk. She jumped, raising both hands as if surrendering, petrified to move at all. Tyler slammed on his brakes and somehow veered around her.

"Jesus Christ!" I shouted. "Are you ever going to learn?" I was shaking.

"I'm sorry. That was really stupid."

"God, we should go back and apologize to that poor woman," I said. But I knew Tyler was too proud. I was really upset at him and hoped he had learned a lesson.

I was also reminded again how fragile life really is. Here I was, going to treatments every day to fight a disease that I had been fighting for a year. Just as that woman could have been killed or maimed, so too could I have been killed crossing the crosswalk to get into Tyler's car that afternoon. It took me about ten minutes to stop shaking, but Tyler seemed to have forgotten it right away.

I wondered whether maybe that was why I had cancer and he didn't. I stressed about things, I felt guilty about things, and I got upset about things. Did I let too much bother me? Would I have been better off it I'd been able to deal with life in a lighter way?

Pondering these questions, I realized that after my experience with cancer, I would never again be able to take life lightly. Life was too short. Life was too fragile. I hoped Tyler would ponder those same questions.

Tyler was a great friend, one of my best, and I hoped that the time he spent in the waiting room and his experience with the pedestrian would affect him. I hoped he would enjoy life as he always had, but I also hoped he wouldn't be stupid, because I was afraid that he might one day hurt himself or someone else. I realized that I loved him. I don't know if I had ever thought about a friend that way before that day.

*   *   *

The next morning was Thursday and I was pretty excited when I woke up. Meeting Carolyn would be a total wildcard. I had no idea what to expect but figured I should be realistic about it. I liked her, but she had mentioned having a boyfriend. I was going to be a gentleman and try to just get to know her better as a friend. Besides, I knew I wasn't her type. She liked punk dudes, and I was about as far from being a punk rocker as you could get.

At lunchtime I walked up to my favorite sandwich shop, bought a tuna-and-olive sandwich, and brought it back to Herman-Justin Plaza outside of the Hyatt Regency near the Embarcadero Building Four plaza. It was a nice day to sit outside and enjoy the sun and the scenery. As I took a bite of the sandwich, I felt a burning sensation across the top of my tongue. The pain was noticeable but not enough to prevent me from finishing my sandwich. After all I'd been through, it would take severe pain to stop me from eating. I assumed that I had a couple of canker sores developing.

After work I headed off to treatment. As luck would have it, the technicians were running a little late. At five after four, I got in for my appointment. I didn't mention anything about my tongue because I figured it was no big deal.

By 4:15, I was finished, so I headed over to the party to look for Carolyn. As I approached the crosswalk, I saw Carolyn in her white nurse's uniform heading toward the same crosswalk only a few feet away. We both noticed each other at the same time.

"Hey, how's it going?" Carolyn said. "Ready to have a cocktail or two tonight?"

"Sure, why not," I replied.

The party was pretty low-key. I got the impression that the medical community at UCSF didn't spend much time at parties. Most of the people there seemed preoccupied. I figured that they probably didn't go to a lot of parties because they were always working. Also, most doctors would never have gotten to where they were if they spent a lot of time partying.

Carolyn saw a few people she knew, but seemed somewhat bored. She suggested that we leave and head over to her house so that she could change. Her apartment was on Cole Street, only about a ten-minute walk. Carolyn wanted to get into something more comfortable and then get a bite to eat. Whatever she felt like doing was fine with me.

When we got to her apartment she showed me around and then turned on some music. We had talked about different bands and we had some common tastes in music, so she suggested that I flip through her albums to see if I saw anything I wanted to play while she changed.

I rummaged through her albums and then stopped to look around her room. Clothes were strewn about, and her bed was unmade. For some reason it didn't surprise me that she was disorganized and sloppy at home, though she was very meticulous, clean, and organized at work.

A moment later she came out of the bathroom wearing a pair of grey cotton pants and a casual top. I had expected her to put on something less mainstream. When she bent down to gather some things from the floor, I couldn't help noticing her beautiful figure.

"Do you mind going on a little drive across town with me first? I just remembered that I need to drop something off at this lady's house. She's been waiting for it for awhile now. It'll just take a minute."

"No problem," I said. If all we did was drive around town that night, that would have been fine with me. It was just nice to have female companionship again.

We chatted comfortably in the car. On the way back, she parked close to Haight Street instead of going back to her apartment. We walked up and down a few streets and then decided to go into a Japanese restaurant.

"You ever had sake before?" she asked me as we walked through the door.

"Yeah, a couple times," I responded. I didn't tell her that I hadn't cared for it.

We asked for a table for two and were seated right away. Carolyn was dying for some appetizers, so I encouraged her to pick whatever she wanted.

After the sake was delivered, Carolyn raised her cup and said "Cheers!"

I tipped my cup to hers and took a sip. It burned like fire. My tongue felt scorched. I didn't want to say anything. I slugged down some water and pretended that everything was fine.

As I ate, I noticed my tongue was burning more and more. I was losing my appetite in a hurry. Carolyn ordered a Sapporo Beer and I joined her. The beer stung as much as the sake.

I sipped my beer like a cup of hot tea. I didn't want to complain and I only hoped that Carolyn wouldn't notice. I enjoyed the conversation but was getting more and more uncomfortable by the moment. I tried to imagine what it would have been like to kiss Carolyn. I was sure that despite the pain in my mouth, I would still be able to muster the strength to kiss her if she were willing.

We walked back to her car and talked about things we never talked about in the hospital. She was a very interesting and open person. We got along great. There was never a moment of silence.

Without discussing what to do next, I quickly realized Carolyn was driving toward the MUNI station to drop me off. I thanked her for a fun night. She quickly wrote her name and home phone number on a piece of paper and handed it to me.

"Let's keep in touch," she said. "We should do this again."

"Ya, I had a great time," I said. "I'll stop by the nurse's station again soon."

As I walked toward the elevator, I filled up with sadness. Carolyn had been nice to me because Carolyn was a nice person. She wasn't interested in me romantically, though. I had to avoid her. I liked her but it was clear I had no chance with her. I knew I couldn't just be a friend with Carolyn. I was too attracted to her to remain only friends. I wasn't going to call her or stop by Fourteen Long again. It would be too painful.

Even though I had a good time with Carolyn and it was a positive experience in many ways, I realized that spending time with women was going to be too difficult. I was deformed, disfigured. No young woman would find me attractive any more.

* * *

I'd been invited to a couple of Christmas parties that weekend and I decided to not show up. Part of me didn't want to deal with all the questions that I would have to answer and another part of me didn't want to deal with women because I knew I couldn't get one interested in me any more. Besides, my mouth was killing me.

The next day at treatment I asked to see a doctor to discuss the burning sensations I was having on my tongue. A doctor I had never met before gave me the first looking over. After examining me for a couple of minutes he suggested that Dr. Palmero take a look.

Dr. Palmero did his own exam and asked me a few questions about what kinds of foods and drinks burned my tongue and which didn't. By then, everything I was eating or drinking stung, even water.

"It looks like thrush to me," he said. He told me that apparently the radiation was killing all the natural bacteria in my mouth and allowing the natural yeast in my mouth to flourish. He gave me some suppositories to suck on but warned me that it could get worse before it got better.

"Great," I replied sarcastically.

He also suggested stopping the radiation treatments until the infection healed, despite the fact that we were only three weeks into the treatment.

"But isn't the whole purpose of radiation to have the treatment every day?" I asked.

"Ideally, yes, but it is okay to take a few days or a week off. We don't really have a choice here. The infection won't go away if we keep administering this to you."

"But when I go back to normal treatments, won't I just get the thrush again?"

"You may and you may not. If you do start showing symptoms again, we might be able to give you the suppositories early on to prevent a full-blown infection. Right now it's pretty full-blown, though."

He told me I could eat and drink whatever felt comfortable. "But you probably won't be able to eat comfortably, so I'd suggest you talk with our nutritionist. There are things you can drink that are high in calories."

Not another nutritionist, I thought. Not that horrible woman from Moffitt again. I prayed that Radiation Oncology had their own nutritionist. Dr. Palmero gave me my prescription and told me to come back to see him at my regular appointment time on Monday. The receptionist escorted me back to an examining room to wait for the nutritionist. A few minutes later, the door opened. It was the witch herself.

'Oh God, no!' I said to myself. I was trapped.

"Hi Terry," she said. "I thought I'd run into you again. How have you been doing?"

We spoke about my surgery and radiation a little bit, and she suggested that I eat puddings, Jell-O, milkshakes and anything that was low in acid. She told me to avoid drinking orange juice altogether. Her advice was solid, though I still would have preferred someone else's help. I thanked her but didn't open the door to any other discussion. She let me get away without a fight. I couldn't believe it. I survived her.

*   *   *

I got home at about six-thirty that night, entirely exhausted. I had been out two nights in a row. I had an infection that was going to make it difficult for me to get my vital nutrients at a time when I needed them the most. I wondered if I had been burning too many candles at one time. I wondered if I would have dodged the infection by staying home and getting more rest, instead of running around chasing a nurse that I had no chance with.

The bottom line was that I had the infection and there was nothing I could do about it. I couldn't blame myself. It wasn't like I had been out drinking into the wee hours of the night. Dr. Zaring had told me I needed to have a little bit of fun, and he was probably right.

"You poor thing," my mother said when I told her. "You've been through so much. Why this?"

I hated it when she said things like that. I had finally resolved that I had no choice but to deal with it, so why question it any more?

My mother drove me down to the store to load up on all the things that I could eat and drink. Then we picked up my suppositories. Mom couldn't refrain from laughing when I told her I had been instructed to suck on the suppositories. "I can't believe he's giving you those, honey. I've used them myself when I had yeast infections. Are you sure it's okay to suck on them?"

"Yes. Dr. Palmero gave me pretty clear instructions." I popped one in my mouth on the drive home. Surprisingly, the suppository was actually soothing to suck on, and the taste wasn't all that bad.

There were only a couple of days before Christmas Day. I was immediately thankful for my Thanksgiving holiday as I realized food and drinks were going to be out of the question for Christmas.

*   *   *

But each day got more uncomfortable. By Sunday I had to stop eating pudding as that began stinging my tongue too. Jell-O and vanilla ice cream and vanilla milkshakes were about all I could handle. The pain got so bad that I had to call the doctor for pain medication.

By Sunday night I was having difficulty speaking because it hurt too much every time my tongue came into contact with my hard palate. I tried to speak by pressing my tongue tightly to the roof of my mouth and holding it there without moving my tongue more than a fraction in any direction.

I called work and mouthed enough words to let them know I couldn't make it in Monday. I told Liz I would check in each day and let her know how I was doing. She was concerned about me and told me not to worry about work. I went back to the clinic Monday afternoon to see the doctor, who decided that I probably needed a whole week off. I was going to miss five treatments. As it turned out, I only missed four days instead of five, because the clinic was closed for the Christmas holiday. I just hoped that there weren't any cells struggling to survive because, if there were, I was giving them a window of opportunity.

I wondered why I was even thinking those thoughts. The time had come for more visualization and positive imaging. I had to make the time to do that, however busy I was getting. Fortunately, I was able to take a few days off at Christmas time to relax and just hang out with my family.

*   *   *

On the morning of Christmas Eve Day my tongue felt so raw that I had to avoid talking altogether. Sleeping seemed to be the only way to avoid the pain. Dr. Palmero had prescribed Dilaudid, a pretty strong painkiller that I could take every four hours, but it didn't really relieve the pain. What it did do was cause drowsiness, and that was okay with me. I knew the more I could sleep the better off I would be.

I fell asleep at about 3:30 and woke three hours later feeling rested, but I knew right away that my tongue felt the same as it had before I went to sleep, as if the butcher had run my tongue through his meat grinder and then reattached it to my mouth.

* * *

I took a notepad and pen out to the family room. While I'd been asleep, a large group of our family friends had arrived for drinks. My hair was sticking straight up in the air and I hadn't shaved in two days. I looked like a complete bum but I felt too sick to care. I had discovered that warm tea with lots of honey in it was very soothing to my tongue. So, while everyone drank scotch, beer and vodka, I had warm tea with honey. The honey felt so smooth and soft on my tongue. I only wished I had discovered it sooner.

Everyone was talking, but after a few minutes I realized how difficult it was to be able to hear but not be able to talk. I tried writing notes in response to comments I was hearing, but the conversation was moving too fast for me to keep up with pen and paper. Finally I slid back into my bedroom to read, and people came in to say hi.

By eight, everyone had left and we sat down to a family dinner. Mom had decided on turkey again, hoping that I'd be able to eat some of the side dishes, but I had resigned myself to Jell-O and vanilla ice cream.

My father said grace and thanked God that we were all together to share Christmas. Rob added thanks that I was able to join everyone for Christmas and that I was clear of my cancer.

It was our tradition to open gifts on Christmas Eve, handing them out one at a time. We sat around and drank a little champagne, shared boxes of candy, and laughed and joked about everything imaginable, including some of the presents. The laughing hurt my tongue, and every once in a while I had to take a break and leave the room. But I realized that laughing was probably the best medicine for anything. It was worth a little pain to get a good laugh.

I finally wrote a little note to Rob and asked him to share it with everyone. On the note I wrote, "Stop joking around. My vagina hurts," referring to my yeast-infected mouth. That shocked everyone, especially my mother. She got over it though. How could I do wrong on that Christmas?

*   *   *

Christmas Day was much like Christmas Eve for me. I felt too sick to go to church. I felt a little guilty about it, but not enough to ask for forgiveness.

The thought of another bowl of vanilla ice cream and another can of Ensure made me feel like throwing up, but I knew I had to keep up my strength. I found that I could sort of plug my nose while I downed the Ensure and that way I didn't have to taste it.

The next day my mouth felt less sore. It was going to be a few more days before I could eat normally again, but certain types of food were easier to eat.

As Dr. Palmero had predicted, I missed four treatments before he felt that the infection had healed enough to put me back on the radiation. Things went well over the next week and my tongue returned to normal. I regained my appetite and I found that I hadn't lost one pound during the entire course of my treatment. I guess all that sugar and fat I had consumed over the Christmas holidays had stored extra calories for me.

*   *   *

I went back to work the week between Christmas and New Year's. I was feeling really good and hadn't noticed any other side effects. On Tuesday I stepped out for lunch and was walking up Market Street a few blocks. The wind was blowing, and my right eye was watering. I blotted my right eye with my index finger. I figured that it was just the wind and didn't think much of it.

But after lunch, when I went back to work, I kept blinking over and over again, trying to clear the blurred vision in my right eye. My eyes had been checked fairly recently, and I knew I had 20/20 vision. I ran to the restroom to look at my eye and felt myself starting to shake.

'Oh, shit,' I thought to myself, 'I hope there aren't cancer cells invading my eye.' I felt around the inside edge of my eye where the scar line remained from surgery. I pressed on it. It felt hard.

'Was it hard before?' I asked myself. 'Do I have a lump or is it just scar tissue?' I tried to calm myself down, to tell myself that the cancer was gone and wasn't coming back. I'd be seeing Dr. Palmero later that afternoon and could ask him to take a look at it. But I couldn't stop worrying. Not only was it hard for me to see things, but I was so anxious that it was hard to concentrate as well.

As soon as I got to the radiation clinic I asked to see Dr. Palmero.

A few moments later, he walked in and greeted me with a friendly smile. "What do you have going on today?"

"I'd like you to take a look at my right eye. I seem to be getting blurred vision, and it keeps tearing up."

"Let's take a look." He pulled out a probe and pressed on the scar line right next to my eye a few times. My eye filled with fluid. He rolled away from me and searched for another instrument, a long syringe. "Put your head back for me and hold steady. I'm going to insert this in your tear duct and try to irrigate it. It might hurt just a little bit. Tell me if you taste some fluid in the back of your mouth after I inject the fluid."

Watching that sharp needle coming close to my eye was terrifying. I braced my hands on the examining table.

'Ouch,' I said to myself, too cool to show any pain. Dr. Palmero tried to inject the fluid into my tear duct, but it ran down my cheek. He quickly handed me a Kleenex to blot my face.

"Sorry about that," he said. "I'm going to try one more time."

The syringe approached my eye one more time and again I clutched at the examining table. Ouch again.

"Did you taste anything?" Dr. Palmero asked.

"No. At least I don't think so," I replied.

"Okay," he said. "Let me tell you what's happening. The radiation has probably sealed up your tear duct, so the tears are backing up. In other words, the tears that drain from your upper tear duct to coat your eye have nowhere to go. They cannot drain out your lower tear duct. You need to see an ophthalmologist who can open it back up. It might close again, but it's worth a try."

I was relieved that he was so sure of himself. I just hoped I wouldn't lose my tear duct permanently. I couldn't imagine having to blot my eye every five minutes. How would I shoot hoops, play golf, or catch fly balls if my right eye were going to blur on me unannounced?

"Do you have an ophthalmologist, or do you need me to recommend one?" Dr. Palmero asked. "If you have your own that is probably better. Opening your tear duct is not a very complicated procedure, so you don't necessarily need to see someone here at UCSF."

I told him that I would call my own ophthalmologist, who was closer to home. I headed back to the waiting room wondering what else the radiation was going to burn or mutilate in my head. I was beginning to realize how very lethal and powerful radiation was.

The next morning I called my ophthalmologist. Fortunately, he was able to see me the following day. The tearing wasn't getting any worse and it wasn't that uncomfortable, but I was afraid if I didn't get the tear duct opened quickly it might shut on me for good.

*   *   *

When I showed up at the ophthalmologists' office I once again had to recount my medical history over the past year. As I described the procedures I had had in such a short period of time, I realized that I really had had a great deal of medical attention, more than most people have in their lifetimes.

The doctor didn't seem surprised by my situation. He listened, wrote down a few notes, and asked me to follow him into his 'procedure' room. He did a few quick eye tests to make sure that my eyes were still in good condition and that the radiation hadn't damaged any element of the eye itself. Then he looked at my tear duct and grabbed a syringe that looked exactly like the kind Dr. Palmero had used.

"Hold on. I'm going to try to push some fluid through the tear duct," he said.

He was far less gentle than Dr. Palmero was. He jammed the syringe into my tear duct forcibly and began rotating it in tiny circles once it was in my tear duct. It felt as if he was stretching it as far as he could in all directions. It hurt like hell.

I tried to hide my discomfort. I held onto the chair with all my strength so I wouldn't budge and end up with the syringe in the middle of my eyeball.

"Anything dripping into the back of your throat?" he asked.

"Not yet," I said, trying to hold every muscle in my face steady.

He pulled out the syringe, fiddled with it, then tried again. I knew that if there had been an earthquake at that instant, I would have lost the eye.

"I taste something," I said at last.

"Good. We finally got through. It looks as if only part of your tear duct is intact. How much more radiation do you have?" he asked.

I told him that I had another eight treatments or so, plus the iridium implants.

"I think it's going to close up again. You're either going to have to come see me regularly to open it up and irrigate it, or we can do a little procedure and put a plastic tube in there. The tube will prevent the tissue from closing up."

"Is it okay to have something plastic in there?"

"Oh, yes. I'd call Dr. Palmero before doing it anyway," he said.

"How extensive a procedure would this be?"

"Oh, we can do it right here in the office. I'll give you a local anesthetic, and it'll probably take about forty-five minutes. I can probably schedule you on Friday."

"Sounds good," I replied. I figured that inserting a little tube through my existing tear duct couldn't be too complicated. I'd been through so much that I forgot to ask for more details.

*   *   *

Dr. Palmero agreed that I should go ahead with the procedure, so I scheduled it for Friday. I took Friday off, afraid of making too many commitments, and not really knowing how I would feel after the procedure.

The doctor's assistant gave me a gown, washed down my face, and applied a topical anesthetic to the area to numb it before the doctor administered the more potent anesthetic.

The injection wasn't too uncomfortable. Seconds later though, the doctor picked up another sharp instrument. I felt pressure against my nose. He seemed to be pushing with a lot of force—so much that I thought he was going to end up piercing my brain. Suddenly, the instrument broke through and I heard a sickening crunch. I felt no pain, but the sound was horrifying.

'What the fuck was this guy doing to me?' I wondered, but I didn't want to ask any questions during the procedure.

The doctor continued to fiddle around with various instruments and finally stepped back and removed his gloves. "All through."

"Is the tube in there?" I asked.

"Yes. I hope it stays in place, but with what you have to work with in that area, I did the best I could. You're missing a lot of bone and tissue around your eye, but I think this will help you."

"What was that crunching sound?"

"I had to break through some bone to create a new opening for the tube. It'll replace your existing tear duct. We might be able to go back later and fix it, but this should solve the problem for now."

The tube did improve things. The tears still collected, but less. The following week, Dr. Palmero wanted to take a look. He stuck his syringe into the new opening, and I immediately tasted the fluid as it ran down the back of my throat.

Dr. Palmero seemed satisfied with the results, and though I wasn't 100% without excess tears blurring my vision, I decided that whatever had been done was good enough.

CHAPTER THIRTEEN

Starts and Stops

Because I still wanted to finish Cal and get my degree, I had re-enrolled for the spring semester. My radiation therapy was supposed to be completed around January 15, and school started January 20.

Radiation Oncology had told me there would be about a week between the completion of my radiation and the iridium implants procedure. I figured I could enroll in classes before going back for the implants.

I had some discussions with my father about medical insurance and he thought it made sense for me to enroll as a part-time student. Under his medical policy, I was covered for my condition as long as I remained a student or until I turned twenty-five. I would have had to remain in school for a very long time to make it to the age of twenty-five, but I figured I could extend my thirty remaining units into two years instead of one.

My father's biggest fear was that I would finish school before my medical treatments were completed and be uninsurable. His company offered great comprehensive coverage, and none of us really knew where my treatment and reconstruction would take me. I was pretty confident that Cravens was going to have me looking like Terry again within the next year, but my father might not have been so sure.

He wanted to play it safe, and he convinced me. I decided to take seven units, only two classes, and work three days a week. One upside was that I was going to be able to save a lot of money. I was already sitting on a government student loan for $2,500 that had come in right after I'd dropped out in the sixth week of the fall semester. I had that stashed in the bank on top of some other scholarships that had come in while I was in the hospital. My fraternity had granted me $1,600 and the Chubb Foundation, an arm of my fathers' company, had given me another $900. I wasn't doing too badly for sitting at home watching television and reading books.

I planned to move back into the fraternity the week before school started. Fortunately, my seniority enabled me to get a single room downstairs, away from all the rowdies. I wanted to live at the house and try to reintegrate myself back into the Greek system, but I also wanted my space. By living downstairs I was able to come and go as I pleased.

I was a little nervous about returning to the Zete house, even though most of my close friends had seen me and talked to me throughout my ordeal. I was hoping to just blend into the surroundings again and not be noticed too much, but people still found ways to locate me. Everyone I saw gave me warm welcomes. I got hugs from some guys and handshakes from others. It was time for my return. I was ready to start living in the real world again. My goal was to try to live as I had before—physically, mentally, and socially.

*　　*　　*

I finished the rest of my radiation treatments without any more complications. I never lost my appetite. I didn't lose any weight, and I never felt very fatigued. The only continuing side effect was the tearing. But that was more an irritant than anything else.

During the last week of treatment, my mother noticed a little bald spot, about two inches high and an inch wide, on the back of my head, a result of the radiation treatment. I went into the bathroom and turned around in front of the mirror, holding a hand-held mirror directly in front of my face. The bald spot wasn't huge, but it was noticeable.

'Shit,' I said to myself. 'How long has that been there? Why didn't anyone tell me sooner?' I was embarrassed all of a sudden, wondering how long I had been walking around with a hole in the back of my head.

I began combing my hair to cover the spot. Fortunately, I had enough hair at that time to cover it. Maybe I'd had that spot for weeks now, but I doubted it.

The bald spot didn't bother me that much, but I did start wondering what else might be happening that I hadn't really noticed. After all, it was my brother, not I, who had first noticed my flared nostril. I decided to take the time to examine myself more thoroughly.

The next morning I brushed my teeth and cleaned my palatal area as always, a task that took about ten minutes to complete. I had to go through a rigorous mouth and teeth-cleaning process three times a day, or after I ate anything between meals. I had been told to spray warm salt water into my mouth and nose to keep the areas clean. I had to fill a syringe with salt water over and over again and irrigate my mouth and nostrils to loosen crusted blood and mucus that built up inside my mouth and nose. Unlike before all the surgery, I couldn't blow my nose with Kleenex to remove mucous buildup. Blowing my nose naturally had become an impossibility.

I finished brushing and popped my denture into my mouth where it fit nice and snug. I then pulled out my shaver and began splashing hot water on my face to open my pores for a closer shave. As I started applying the shaving cream to my cheeks and upper lip, I noticed there were very few hairs left on my upper lip. I had been shaving the area every day, and, probably because shaving was just an exercise of habit, hadn't even noticed that the shadow of hair on my upper lip had all but vanished. All that remained were a few visible roots. I thought about my bald spot. Of course—if the hair on the back of my head was gone, it would make sense for the hair to be gone on the front of my head since the radiation beam was being directed at my front side.

Once again, I was amazed that I hadn't noticed another change to my face. There were barely any signs left of facial hair on my upper lip. As I looked closer, I realized that the lack of facial hair was one more characteristic of my appearance that had been altered. I looked even more deformed without a shadow on my lip. I had a heavy shadow of facial hair everywhere else. I looked like Abraham Lincoln—a heavy beard and no mustache. I decided that I had to shave every day and on weekends, or I would have one more abnormality that people would be able to identify. At that very moment it occurred to me that one way I could hide some of my facial scars would be to grow a mustache. I didn't have scars that a beard would cover, but a mustache would cover up a lot. All I could do was wait and see.

*   *   *

Being back at the Zete House had presented a few complications right off the bat. All my closest friends wanted to go out drinking the first night I got back. What could I say? I didn't want to be a wimp and say no. But I also knew that I had more treatment ahead of me, and I wanted to remain as strong as I could by getting plenty of rest and not abusing my body.

That first night John tried to convince me to go to Kip's, a pizza and beer restaurant on Durant Way. I didn't mind going out and eating dinner over a couple of beers, but I knew by going with John that it would lead to more than a couple of beers.

As we headed to Kip's I realized that I didn't miss the partying all that much. I wasn't looking forward to a night on the town as much as I had looked forward to just living normally. But I was also focused on getting well and strong again. Getting my strength back was the most important thing to me. Drinking to excess would do me no good. I didn't need to get drunk to have a good time. Maybe I had changed a little bit.

Had the cancer made me a more responsible person? Had I grown up all of a sudden? Did it take cancer to make me realize that there was more to life than partying every night?

* * *

Fortunately, I didn't get too much pressure on those first few nights back to stay out until the wee hours of the morning. My friends understood what I was going through. They just wanted me to have a good time again. And they wanted to share in those good times.

One of the things I realized in those first few days back to school was that my friends outside of the fraternity were hanging out with some of my friends in the fraternity. I was glad to see that my friends' visits to UCSF had created some new friendships and formed some new bonds, partially on account of my hospitalization. It was great to see some of my old high school buddies hanging out with my fraternity buddies.

My observation awakened me to the importance of staying in touch with friends. I had to make a better effort in the future. Having a support structure seemed so vital to everyday life. I hadn't realized that until I was in a time of need. I recognized that everyone had problems, whether they were physical, mental or emotional, and the close friends we had were the ones who helped us get through those times.

Many people I never expected to hear from came out of the woodwork. Acquaintances called me and came to see me. I found out I had more friends than I had realized. Then I thought about Kerri. I still hadn't heard from her and I had considered her to be one of my best friends. She was the only real surprise.

*   *   *

Enrolling in only two classes and selecting only one upper division course made it pretty easy to get the schedule I wanted. I still hadn't completed English 1B, the second and final English requirement needed to graduate. My other class was on Eastern European Politics, a class I figured would be interesting and one that would give me three more units toward fulfilling my major.

I bought my books right away for a change. The first essay assigned for English 1B was suppose to be on assorted Ernest Hemingway short stories. The paper was due the following Monday, so I figured I would read the short stories in the hospital while my iridium implants baked away at the roof of my mouth.

I told a few friends that I was heading back to the hospital for a two-day treatment, but asked them to keep it quiet. I didn't want people speculating that I was already having problems and had to be readmitted to the hospital. I left Berkeley and headed home in my Ford Falcon. Mom was going to take me to the hospital the next morning. Since I couldn't have many visitors, I brought plenty of extra reading and figured on watching a lot of CNN to catch up on the news of the world.

I was scheduled for an appointment with both Dr. Palmero and Dr. Corria. They were going to examine me and then get me fitted with the iridium-laced obturator.

Dr. Zaring, the maxillofacial prosthetics specialist, had to make me a new obturator the week before so that my existing one could be sent to radiology and fitted with the iridium seeds. Obviously, the iridium-laced obturator would be destroyed after the treatment was complete. What seemed amazing to me was that the new obturator was considered a temporary as well. Dr. Zaring figured my mouth would change quite a bit over the ensuing months due to decreased swelling and possible reconstruction that could alter the cavity around my existing palate.

I tried to estimate what the cost would be for all the obturators, knowing that my permanent obturator would cost around

$3,500. The temporaries that had been made and all the adjustments Dr. Zaring had to make to them must have been adding up. I laughed to myself as I recalled my parents telling me how fortunate I was that I never needed braces. They used to remind me how lucky I was that I had good, healthy, straight teeth. I had never had a cavity either.

Arriving at UCSF, I was pretty fired up for the final leg of my radiation treatment. The doctors were satisfied that all looked well from their examination of me. Dr. Corria then took me down the hallway to meet a technologist for the fitting.

I was taken to a small room in the far corner of the Radiation Oncology Clinic and seated in an examining chair. The room was full of heavy metal objects on wheels. I had no idea what any of the equipment was designed to do.

A middle-aged, kind of pudgy but enthusiastic guy, who turned out to be the technologist, met us in the examining room. He was wearing a jump suit that looked like he was heading off to space. I assumed it had to have been a hazardous materials protective suit of some kind.

The technologist quickly described how the iridium "seeds" had been implanted into my obturator. He cautioned me that I was going to be exposed to a fair amount of radiation over the 48-hour period and for that reason visitors would not be allowed to see me. He comforted me by saying that even though others weren't suppose to have a lot of contact with me, I wasn't receiving a dangerous amount of radiation. He threw out some comparisons to x-rays and other things we are commonly exposed to, all the while gesturing wildly with his hands.

"What I want to do is fit you with this obturator down here first to make sure it is okay. That way if we need to make adjustments we can take care of it now." He then handed me an x-ray blanket and asked that I place it over my stomach and abdomen.

Then it occurred to me that the blanket was going to be a fixture for two days. "Is there a risk of sterilization with these iridium implants?" I asked.

He moved his head lower, toward mine, and holding out his hands as if to show a measurement, said, "No. Actually it makes everything huge down there." He started laughing wildly. He thought that was pretty funny.

I laughed too, but I did want a sincere answer to my question.

"No, really," I said. "Is there a risk?"

"No, not really," he responded. "It would take a ton of constant exposure to pose a real risk. The blanket just shields the radiation to a greater degree."

The obturator seemed to fit fine. He then removed it and inserted it back into a large stainless steel drum that sat on wheels and resembled a giant vacuum cleaner. He asked us to follow him down the hall to another room. He wheeled the "stainless steel vacuum cleaner" down the hallway. He unlocked another door and asked me to step inside. I sat down and he again inserted the obturator in my mouth. Insuring that I was comfortable with how it fit, he then grabbed something off the shelf and said, "Let's go!"

Dr. Corria and my mother followed several paces behind the two of us as we headed toward what appeared to be a limited-use elevator. The technologist wanted to escort me to the eleventh floor of Long Hospital by using the least populated hallways and elevators so as to limit the exposure of my implants to other hospital personnel and possible patients.

As we reached the eleventh floor, considered the Cancer Therapy floor of the hospital, we saw people milling around.

"Clear the way!" he shouted, loudly, but in a friendly way. "We have a radioactive patient here!"

The people ahead quickly cleared out of our way by heading into doorways and other patient rooms. I started laughing as I thought how ridiculous my parade must have looked and sounded to people unfamiliar with my type of procedure. I turned around to check on my mother and Dr. Corria trailing behind by about twenty paces. Walking that far behind me was the last thing in the world my mother wanted to do. She would have preferred to be with me and expose herself, but the instructions from Dr. Corria were pretty clear.

"Clear away! Radioactive patient!" the technologist repeated, as we encountered more staff up ahead.

He seemed to be having fun leading the parade. He was laughing and seemingly having a good time. I turned around again to look at my mother. We were both laughing at the spectacle I had somehow become the focal point of.

Finally, we reached my room. I was asked to lie down on top of my bed while Dr. Corria went to the nurse's station to check me in. The technologist followed me into the room.

I dropped my bag down next to the nightstand and then carefully sat down on the bed, afraid of jarring my obturator. I twisted around and lay down on my back. The technician then propped the x-ray blanket over my stomach and groin.

"Remember," he said, "these implants are going to make your penis huge!" He laughed, throwing his hands up toward his shoulders.

A few minutes later Dr. Corria returned with the head nurse and my mother. My mother was asked to stand at the door while Dr. Corria and the nurse entered the room. My bed had a partition on the side facing the door which the technologist had told me was to protect the medical staff from the radiation when they spoke or tended to me. My mother hadn't been allowed in because she didn't have a Geiger counter. All the medical staff on that floor had Geiger counters attached to their hips that enabled them to track the amount of x-rays they were receiving. The nurse explained that I would be fed at regularly scheduled times, but that I wouldn't really have much interaction with the nursing staff unless I needed something. I would be more or less "in isolation" for the entire 48 hours.

I thanked the nurse and assured her that I had plenty of reading to keep me busy. Dr. Corria told me she would stop in occasionally to check on me. Then they turned to head toward the door.

I propped myself up on the bed to get a glimpse of my mother. I waved and told her to go ahead home. "Thanks for taking me. I guess I will see you in a couple days. Check with the nurse's station to find out when you can come back to pick me up."

"Okay, honey. Gosh, I'm sorry you have to sit in here all by yourself for two days," Mom said.

"Oh, I'll be all right. Don't worry about me. This is the easy part," I replied.

It was hard for her to go, but I finally convinced her that she wouldn't be very comfortable standing in the hallway.

Then the technologist said goodbye and headed toward my mother at the door to my room. He pulled out a large spool of yellow tape and said, "I'm sealing you off," laughing all the while as he draped the tape across my open door.

On the tape it read "WARNING." I had warning tape draped across the entrance to my door, much like the tape you see at a dangerous construction zone.

"Well," I thought to myself as I looked at the warning tape, "if I don't have cancer now, I will probably have it in the future." Seeing the warning tape made me realize how curing *and* dangerous radiation could be, all at the same time.

* * *

I spent the afternoon sitting and reading and fidgeting a lot. What I was finding to be the most difficult aspect of the treatment was that, though I felt fine, I couldn't get out of bed to walk around. I felt like I was going to go stir crazy. The technician might as well have strapped my hands and feet to the bedposts so I wouldn't even be tempted to get up and walk around.

I was told to use the restroom as I needed, however the technologist had warned me not to put my head between or close to my knees when I sat on the toilet. You can guess why. My private parts "would grow faster than a watermelon in the summer."

I really wasn't aware that I had a designated nurse that afternoon until my evening nurse walked into my room to introduce herself.

Claire had a very soft, sweet voice. She had soft, milky white skin and dark eyebrows and short dark hair. She was very cute in the way she smiled, but more beautiful when she was expressionless and just listening. I couldn't believe how lucky I had been to be cared for by an entourage of pretty, young nurses.

Claire told me the cancer therapy floor operated on twelve-hour shifts and that she was on duty until 6:00 a.m.. She began to ask me all about myself, seeming to be very interested in finding out who the real person was in "warning tape" room number one.

I told her that I was a senior at U.C. Berkeley but had just re-enrolled after dropping out the prior semester due to all the surgery I had had.

"You go to Cal?" she asked. "Are you in a fraternity there?"

"I am in the Zete House, which is on Bancroft, across from Boalt Hall, the Law School." I explained where it was, thinking she might not have even heard of the house.

"Do you know Tom Biehl?" she asked, smiling and hopeful.

"Ya, I know Tom Biehl. He is one of my older brothers' really good friends."

"Well, I went to high school with Tom. His girlfriend, Laura, is a really close friend of mine. We went to San Diego State together."

"I know Laura. She's hilarious. You probably know Carrie and Mary too, right? Laura, Carrie and Mary were always over at our house once they transferred up to San Francisco State."

"Ya, I know Carrie and Mary. They're a lot of fun."

I wanted to continue talking to Claire, but I was worried about her hanging over my bed panel. I didn't feel right talking to her and knowing my radiation was spilling into her 'space'.

"You better go," I said nicely, bringing my hands to my face to signify the danger of my radiation to her.

"I have a Geiger counter on. It's okay. I will leave when I have to. Unless, of course, you want me to leave?"

"No, no. I just don't want to expose you to all this stuff," I said.

We talked a little more and then she said she had to check on some other patients. She had been in my room talking for about thirty minutes.

As she exited my room, I rose my head up over the panel of my bed to see her go. She was about 5'5" tall, and, despite her nurse's uniform, I could tell she had a nice, firm body. As I lay back down on my bed I wondered if I was just getting desperate or if the UCSF nurses truly were that attractive. Looking back, they were all very pretty. I was the luckiest cancer patient in the world.

*　　*　　*

The next morning was January 27, 1986. I turned on "Good Morning America" and watched the news. I was excited that I would be able to watch the first American civilians go into space on the Challenger Space Shuttle.

As many of us so vividly remember, that ill-fated launch was so very brief. I can remember Tom Brokaw ad-libbing right after the explosion, speculating that the falling debris might have been parachutes. His hopeful words were just that. We quickly found out that the debris was just debris. I had watched the program preceding the launch and had learned all about the mother and school teacher who would be the first female civilian in space. She was so happy and optimistic about her selection and the opportunity ahead of her.

The shock I felt was tremendous. Once again, I realized how fragile life was. People full of life and hope seconds before the crash were suddenly gone forever. Worse was thinking about the aftermath. I prayed quickly for the families and the children left behind.

Claire was off duty when the tragedy occurred, so I had no one to share the experience with. I never really saw the nurse that relieved Claire. I guess she just figured I would press my help button if I needed anything.

*   *   *

Shortly after Claire's shift began she checked on me. She was fairly busy until about 9:00 p.m. with other patients and then she returned to my room. We must have talked for at least an hour. Her Geiger counter never went off, so I didn't bug her to leave. That evening, when she left me to go to sleep, she grabbed one of my hands with both of hers and held it.

As she held my hand tightly she said, "You are a very strong person, Terry. You're going to be fine." She was very serious as she spoke. She then released my hands and said with a big smile, "Come by and say hi next time you're here seeing your doctor."

"I definitely will. Thanks for everything Claire. You made these last forty-eight hours bearable. I really do appreciate it."

"Well, not all my patients are normal and nice like you are. A lot of them are really negative and bitter and it is sometimes hard to try to talk to them."

We said good-bye. As she left the room, I realized I had fallen in love with another nurse. I never asked her if she had a boy-friend or if she was married, because I really didn't want to know. I guess by me not knowing whether or not she was attached left a little hope that I had a chance with Claire. The problem was, I had no plan of action. I was lacking the confidence in myself to ask anyone out. If she said no, I would instantly assume it was because she wasn't attracted to me, not because she may have had someone special in her life. I wasn't prepared to handle rejection yet.

Regardless, I went off to sleep with hopefulness. I was content. Claire had made the forty-eight hour somewhat dreaded treatment episode an enjoyable experience.

The next morning a couple of my doctors checked on me to make sure I wasn't having any problems. Then, when my forty-eight hours was up, my favorite technologist appeared with his vacuum cleaner-like device to carry away my iridium-laced obturator.

I had been warned that I might get burned by the iridium and develop blisters on the roof of my mouth. My mother worried that the treatment would place me back into the world of purees and milkshakes again. But, when the iridium obturator was removed and the new obturator put in its place, I had not noticed any immediate changes or side effects from the treatment. I was glad they had prepared me for it, but happier that I hadn't developed any blisters. Dr. Corria was pretty confident that morning that if I hadn't developed any blistering by then, I probably was not going to develop blisters later.

The warning tape was removed from my door and I was suddenly a free man again. I was free to walk up and down the halls, but best of all, I was free of all my treatment. I was ecstatic, though I didn't want to show it. I wanted to appear strong and confident instead, as if I never had any doubts I would finish the treatment in good health and high spirits. In only a few months I had planned to begin the process of reconstruction so that I could become Terry again.

As I left the hospital to head back to my parents house for the night, I realized that I no longer could use my treatment as an excuse, either to myself or to others. I had come to appreciate having that excuse in my back pocket if for any reason I needed it to turn in an assignment late. Having a valid excuse always made things a little less stressful. The excuse card was something I was fortunate to be able to play if necessary. As far as using the excuse to others, I had to learn to be honest and just say no when I wasn't interested or up to doing something with someone. If I didn't want to go out drinking, I had to tell the truth, which was that I just didn't want to. I no longer could use the excuse that because of my treatment I shouldn't be drinking.

*   *   *

The next morning I drove off to Berkeley to attend my classes, already into the second week.

I hadn't noticed the prior week, but as I entered the room to attend my Political Science 141C class, I spotted Kerri across the room. Fortunately, we hadn't made eye contact, so I quickly turned up the next row of desks and found a seat. I didn't know what to say to her. I had too much pride to approach her. I felt it was her duty to take the initiative.

When class was over I nonchalantly exited the room, clearly giving Kerri an opportunity, if she spotted me, to catch up to me and say hello. I did not turn around and after exiting the building I knew she had left via another route.

Two days later on the way to the same class Kerri and I ran into each other outside of the building.

"Hey Healey," Kerri said, as if she had seen me only the day before.

"Hey Kerri," I replied, in the same tone of voice she had used.

It was as if nothing had happened and no time had elapsed since I had last seen her in October. We didn't hug, though I could have just as easily taken the initiative to hug her. I let her dictate the meeting.

After a couple of minutes of no-content discussion, Kerri inquired about my health. She didn't apologize for not calling or writing, however. She was the only person that had disappointed me. I had thought she was one of my best friends. Now that we had finally met up again, I was even more disappointed.

I began to wonder if a family member of hers had died of cancer or had cancer and perhaps that was why she was having difficulty dealing with me. Did I remind her of something terribly painful?

I wanted to forgive her and forget the past, but I couldn't. Then I asked myself how I would have dealt with it if things were totally reversed, and she was the one with cancer. I hoped that I would have been there for her. But would I have? I will never know. I knew I had to forgive her. It was water under the bridge. It would take time to forgive her, though I knew time would never allow me to forget. I was saddened by the thought that our relationship would probably always be scarred by what had happened.

*   *   *

Back at the Zete House, I ran into Todd, a younger guy who, despite having a bit of an ego, was generally a nice guy.

Todd was standing with about three other guys in the hallway downstairs, and a couple of girls were chatting next to them. The girls I had seen before, but didn't know them. As I headed toward the group, Todd asked loudly, "Hey, Healey. How's the cancer?" His tone of voice was the same as someone would use to ask how your jog had been moments after you finished. It was asked in a manner that typically was responded to positively and with enthusiasm. The girls turned toward me as Todd addressed me.

My instant reaction to myself was to say, "Hey, Todd. My cancer is great, you fucking asshole! It's growing like a weed!" But instead I thought about his question for a moment and tried to withhold my emotions. I decided it would be better to forgive his brashness and be honest.

"Hey, Todd. I'm doing great. I just finished all my treatment and everything looks good."

He didn't know much about my cancer and assumed that I had some form of cancer like leukemia or non-Hodgkin's lymphoma.

"So is it in remission or what?" Todd asked, as everyone else listened, though uncomfortably.

"No, Todd. I'm cured. My cancer is gone. I had a localized tumor. It was totally removed and there are now no signs of it."

"Really?" he smiled. "That's great Terry. It's really amazing what has happened to you."

I refrained from responding to his last comment and continued walking toward my room, telling him I had a phone call to make. The guy had no tact. He had no idea how rude he was being.

I would find that over the next few months I would have many uncomfortable encounters. Almost everyone I saw for the first time after my return had some reaction, though usually it was only in his or her facial expression. Rarely did people say things that they would possibly regret later. Unfortunately, it was the rare occasions that didn't seem so rare at the time, that left an indelible mark on my psyche.

Though people didn't purposely say things to hurt me, the comments had a tremendous impact on my self-esteem and confidence. With each occurrence I climbed deeper into a shell, shielding myself from those that could hurt me with their words. Sometimes what hurt the most were the comments that other people made behind my back that I heard about from my close friends. I wished I had never heard some of those comments.

One thing I heard shortly after my return was a comment another guy in my fraternity had made in front of several guys at the house, many of whom were my friends. What I was told was that Jimmy had said something to the effect that if it were him who had what I had he would have either lived in a closet or hung himself.

Did I really look that horrible that my life would no longer be worth living? I certainly didn't feel that way, but it hurt me tremendously to know that others felt that way.

One evening, a group of us had gone down to the Kingfish for some clam chowder and decided to stay and have pitchers of beer. As typically happens at the Kingfish, students drop in and out throughout the evening to have a beer or two.

I was sitting at a table with my buddies Tyler, John and Rich. Rich's brother Ted strolled in, saw us playing quarters, and decided to participate in the game.

It was my turn. Typically, new players get harassed and forced to drink more shots in order that they catch up to the rest of the players. Ted had seen me only moments prior drinking out of the cup in the center of the table. I bounced the quarter off the table and sunk it into the cup. I turned and pointed my elbow to Ted, the proper way of selecting whom you wanted to drink.

Ted picked up the cup, looked at it and asked me, "Is that contagious? Is what happened to your face contagious, dude?" he asked, peering at my nose and eye, not an expression of humor found anywhere on his face.

I laughed, assuming he was only joking. After all, how stupid can one be? How many twenty-one year olds don't know that cancer isn't contagious? As I chuckled, I noticed Ted was not laughing back. He was still holding the glass in front of him.

I decided not to embarrass him, as shocked as I was. "No, Ted. Cancer is not contagious," I said, giving him the benefit of the doubt that perhaps he didn't know I had cancer, though that would have been hard to believe, given that his brother Rich was one of my best friends.

Satisfied that I would tell him the truth, Ted then tipped the cup back and drained it down his throat. Afterwards, he acted as if nothing had happened. He was all smiles and ready for the next drink. As I tried to concentrate on making the next shot, I couldn't help but think about Ted's question. It opened up an entirely new anxiety that up to now I had never even considered. Would people think I had some horrible, contagious disease that they could catch if they got too close to me or if they drank out of the same glass?

*   *   *

As much as comments like those made me want to climb deeper into my shell, I knew developing a harder shell was what was necessary. I had to block those things out. I couldn't let those types of comments influence my behavior. I knew I had to ignore them and move on. But I also knew that was easier said than done.

A couple of weeks later Tyler, Tom and I went to a dance club out in Danville called Fat Fannies.

As the three of us waded through the maze of people, up ahead Tyler saw a familiar face that happened to be one of the cocktail waitresses. As I tried to catch up to Tyler, I heard the waitress cheerily say, "Hey, Tyler. How's it going?"

"Pretty good, Gwen. How are you?" Tyler asked as she welcomed him with a big hug. Gwen was a friend of Tyler and mine from high school.

As Gwen stepped back from her hug with Tyler, she turned her head toward me. "Hi Gwen," I said nicely. Her eyes widened like huge saucers and she put her right hand over her mouth.

"Oh my God!" she said at me, and quickly turned around and went in the other direction. It was clear that she knew exactly who I was. I guess seeing me differently was too much of a shock for her to take. I was hurt. I looked at Tyler.

"What a bitch!" I said. "I guess she's not even going to help us with drinks."

Tyler was speechless. He didn't know what to say to me. He knew I was upset.

"Fuck her, Terry. She's worthless," Tyler said, in an attempt at consoling me.

I didn't want to ruin the night for Tom and Tyler, but she had wiped out my interest in staying at Fat Fannies. My buddies knew it. I didn't have to tell them. Tyler suggested we leave the bar and go somewhere else. Tom and I followed without questioning why.

We got into Tom's car and headed to Elliot's, a local Danville bar. It was the kind of place you could have a beer and not feel self-conscious, no matter who you were or what you looked like.

* * *

I was trying hard to build a thicker shell around myself but I was also desperately looking forward to having some reconstruction. I figured that anything Dr. Cravens could do would help. I knew as hard as I tried to ignore the comments and reactions about my face, it would always be tough for me. But Dr. Cravens said he would get me back to Terry. I still believed him.

CHAPTER FOURTEEN

Reconstruction . . . Finally

By late March, Dr. Cravens informed me that I could begin reconstruction, which would require three separate surgeries. His goal was to improve the symmetry of my face. However, this time I didn't hear him say he'd get me back to Terry.

I didn't talk to other doctors about reconstruction. All the other doctors and nurses had told me that Dr. Cravens was the best there was. I trusted them because they had seen his work. Also, I figured he knew what there was to work with better than anyone else.

*   *   *

I had high expectations for the first surgery. Cravens hadn't promised much the day before the surgery, but I still anticipated that the outcome would be like the difference between night and day. When I came out from under the anesthetic, I was extremely excited. I couldn't wait to see myself in the mirror. The recovery-room nurse told me the surgery had been successful and that there was a big improvement. The expectation was that Dr. Cravens would focus the procedure around removing the excess tissue from my upper lip and right cheek, as well as creating more structure to my nose. The procedure was to last about four hours and would require at least one night in the hospital.

As soon as I could I walked into my hospital room bathroom, not even thinking to stop and prepare myself for disappointment. I hadn't even considered that the surgery wouldn't be up to my expectations.

I hurried into the bathroom and looked into the mirror above the sink. My jaw dropped. Cravens had thinned the fatty tissue from my shoulder that had been transplanted to my upper lip and cheek area. But that was the only visible change! It was noticeable to me, but the average person would still see a patch of discolored skin pasted onto a nose that was missing virtually an entire nostril. My right ala—the outside wing of my nostril— was still missing, as was the columella, the tissue that separates the two nostrils. My heart sank. I'd told my friends that Cravens was going to rebuild my nose, but obviously I had a long road ahead.

The doctor had warned me that he had to be conservative in the reconstruction process. Because of the radiation treatments, I was susceptible to infection. Also, live-tissue transplants would be far riskier because the radiation had probably permanently limited the blood supply in the radiated areas. Without ample blood supply, skin grafts, bone grafts and cartilage grafts would not necessarily take. I was disappointed. Getting me back to Terry wasn't going to be as easy as I had thought. Cravens seemed to be giving me more and more reasons why my particular case was going to be a difficult one. Why had he been so confident earlier? Had he not realized how much radiation I would receive? Had he been trying to keep me feeling optimistic? I had a lot of questions, but I was also looking forward to the second procedure. After all, the first operation had been kind of preliminary. Cravens told me that he planned to work on rebuilding my ala and columella in the next procedure, six weeks later. I was still confident about my prospects.

But either because of the radiation treatments or because

the defect on the right side of my face was really just composed of fatty tissue covering up a giant hole, my face began to contract toward the defect in all directions. My upper lip began to pull upward toward the defect, and the right side of my nose began to turn slightly in that direction as well. Also, the orbit of my right eye and my right eyelid began to droop downward, making my eyes look asymmetrical. Until then, both eyes had been the same shapes, and the lower eyelids had been at the same level. Things were starting to look so much different.

The cancer surgery was over. I thought my scars had healed. But as I would learn more and more, healing takes a long time. I hoped time would make everything look better, but now I was beginning to think that time was making everything look worse. Time seemed to be both my friend and my enemy. Time would dictate my curability, but it would also affect my appearance—in ways I couldn't predict.

When Cravens saw me again to prepare for the next procedure, I began to realize the severity of my defect. He told me he would try to make my face look as symmetrical as possible but that it would take many surgical steps to give me the structure and the foundation before the real "plastic surgery" could begin.

Although he appeased me by suggesting that he pull some original right cheek tissue over the discolored flap tissue, he also told me he needed new lining tissue to graft inside my right nostril and inside my palate. He planned to take another skin graft from my thigh, the left thigh this time, and more ear cartilage to prop up my drooping right eye and flattened nasal areas.

I had the utmost confidence in Cravens and wasn't going to argue with whatever he felt was necessary. He knew that I wanted to look the way I had before all the cancer surgery.

Some of the cartilage inside my nose failed to take, but the palatal graft was successful. From a medical standpoint, the next two procedures were considered successful. But from an outside observer's point of view, the procedures accomplished very little.

Finally Cravens told me that my condition might require far more reconstruction than he had anticipated. He suggested that we wait before attempting any major reconstruction, such as additional full-thickness skin grafts. The radiation treatments appeared to be causing the transplanted flap tissue to reabsorb. He suggested that I might not have enough tissue around my nose to reestablish the facial symmetry we were striving for, and he began describing other options, such as borrowing muscle and tissue from the back of my head or from my forehead. These full-thickness skin grafts, which would resemble the skin graft I'd had dangling from my chest to my face, were intended to develop a new blood source at the site. And of course, every procedure would require additional surgical steps as well. He even mentioned grafting hipbone into my cheek and other horrible-sounding scenarios. The procedures he described seemed worse than the original ones I'd had in October.

Cravens also told me that it would be better to wait a year or more before undergoing any major reconstructive surgery because the resorption of tissue from the radiation and the healing from the surgery would continue to affect the area for quite some time. Also, the contracting of the tissue around the defect might continue, and that would complicate the reconstruction. And finally, the risk that the cancer could recur after reconstruction would be devastating and wasteful. The confident Dr. Cravens that I had become so accustomed to was starting to sound uncertain. My hopes and dreams of becoming Terry Healey again suddenly vanished. I had thought that the three reconstructive procedures would make everything symmetrical again. They had been carried out—but what had gone wrong? Had it all been just a smokescreen to keep my spirits up? At that point in my life, I wasn't assertive enough to ask Cravens what had changed. He had saved my life. In my mind, he was the one doctor at the Tumor Board who had been willing to take the risks involved in saving me. To me, he was God. But now, suddenly and without warning, he was talking about massive reconstructive procedures that I had never considered or even heard him mention before. I heard amazing stories about people who had been totally reconstructed and brought back to the way they looked before.

Why was my case becoming so difficult?

I didn't know the answer. But if Cravens wasn't going to work on me for another year, I assumed that meant I would have to wait. He knew how badly I wanted the reconstruction and would have recommended someone else to me if he thought it was possible for someone else to do it. But I was beginning to understand that my case was more difficult and more complicated than most. I had to wait until Cravens made the next move. I didn't know what else to do.

"So, we just wait for awhile, ha?" I asked the doctor, seemingly dumbfounded by the exchange we'd just had.

"Well, Terry, there's not much else we can do." He didn't apologize for leading me on earlier.

There was nothing left to say. I put my head down, looked at the floor momentarily, and said, "So, you'll just monitor my situation for the next few months before we schedule anything, right?"

"That's all we can do, Terry. Now, let's hope that Cal team wins a few more games this year, ha?" he chided, trying to steer my attention elsewhere.

We shook hands, but I was speechless. How was I going to continue to face the world every day? I was going to spiral into a depression if something positive didn't happen quickly.

I got into my car and looked in the mirror at myself. I looked ugly. I looked deformed. No girl would want to date me. I was only twenty-one and I wondered if I would ever have a girlfriend again. What the hell was I going to do?

*   *   *

Over the next couple of months I tried desperately to get back into the swing of things. I forced myself to go to parties and pushed myself to go out to dinner and bars with friends. I knew I had to learn to live with my disfigurement. I didn't know how long I would look this way. I figured that in two years I would probably look pretty good again, but in the meantime I had to try to learn to live with myself the way I was.

I learned that staying busy was the best medicine. The more activities and goals I could coordinate at the same time, the less time I spent being preoccupied with my face. As soon as Cravens gave me the go-ahead, I went back to a vigorous running and exercise routine.

I wanted to get back into shape so that I would feel better about myself. I focused on running and weightlifting, figuring I could strengthen, tone, and build muscle while I was also building my heart rate back up. I had missed running more than anything else—being outside and breathing fresh air were things I no longer wanted to take for granted. I liked not only the high I got from running, but also the tremendous cleansing feeling I felt from all the sweating. The weightlifting restored some of the confidence I had lost. I wanted to look good in clothes. If I couldn't feel good about my face, I wanted to feel good about my body.

*   *   *

That summer, after the semester ended, my friend Tyler and I agreed to housesit at our friend Dave's parents' house in Danville, while they built their new home in Idaho. We lived in the guesthouse but had access to the pool and tennis court. The house was also close to the base of Mt. Diablo, a 3,500-foot mountain that was great for mountain-bike riding and hiking.

My twenty-second birthday was August 18. I wanted a low-key celebration, so my brothers invited me over for a barbecue at Brian's house. As I pulled my Toyota Landcruiser up his steep driveway, I decided I would park in the gravel next to his backyard fence. As I bent down to put the parking brake on, I looked over the fence and saw a line of guys filling beer cups from a keg. I'd been fooled—it was a surprise birthday party. I was actually excited. There were a couple of girls, but only one of them was a friend of mine—Kerri, of all people. I was stunned.

I was happy that she had made the effort to come all the way from Oakland. This time when we saw each other, it was all smiles.

"Healey, how are you?" she asked cheerily. Finally the ice was broken between us.

"I'm great, Kerri. Thanks for coming out here for this." I hugged her and asked where all the other girls from our group were. Everyone was busy but Kerri. Suddenly, Kerri was looking like a friend who was making a great effort.

But Kerri shone in party situations like these. She could hang around a keg with guys better than any girl I knew could.

After dinner, we began playing quarters. Kerri was standing behind me. She didn't want to play because she knew she had to drive home. I respected that. I also thought she looked really cute that night. I continued to sink the quarters in the cup on the table. I couldn't miss.

"Pretty hot, Healey," Kerri said. "You're a stud, dude!"

I got bold. "I have a deal for you Kerri," I said. "If I make five in a row, I get to kiss you."

"You'll never hit five in a row!"

"Is it a deal or what?"

"Okay. Let's see it."

I felt a hint of interest from her smile as she spoke to me. Though I didn't know for sure if she was still interested in me, I figured I would find out soon enough, and I knew I could hit five in a row. I made the next shot. I pointed my elbow at Brian to drink. I made the next shot. I pointed my elbow at Tyler to drink. I hit the next two shots. Then I looked up at Kerri.

"Here it is. Number five, here we go!" I bounced the quarter on the table and it dropped directly into the cup. I pointed my elbow at Kerri and said, "Drink up!"

She gulped down the shot. "What can I tell you—you're a stud, Healey."

I got out of my chair and stood in front of her feeling very confident. "I earned my kiss," I said.

I walked her into the family room away from everyone else and we kissed a few times. I wanted to go a little further but she stopped me. It wasn't right. Nothing was right about us being together that night. I was half-drunk but was still sober enough to understand what she was telling me, and I didn't feel totally rejected. I respected her. She wasn't going to give out to me because she felt sorry for me or because she still liked me. The situation had to be right or it wasn't going to happen.

Finally we went back to the rest of the gang. I sat back down and immersed myself into the quarter's game and Kerri carried on conversations with others in the room until she finally left, sober and respected by all.

The next morning, I felt horrible in more ways than one. I was hung over, but I felt even worse about making the move on Kerri. I hadn't been with a girl in so long and I wanted to remember what it was like. But I knew that morning that I couldn't really be with Kerri seriously. There had been too much history between us. We just needed to try to keep our friendship together. As soon as I had a chance, I called her.

"Hi. I know you probably don't want to talk to me, but I wanted to apologize for last night."

"Healey, don't even worry about it. It was no big deal. You don't have to say sorry."

That was one of the things I liked so much about Kerri. She took everything so lightly. If she said it was no big deal to her, then I knew it was no big deal.

We talked for a few minutes about the party and then said good-bye. As I hung up the phone, I thought about the irony that she had forgiven me for what I had done, but I still hadn't totally forgiven her for not being there for me when I was sick. Maybe deep down I'd tried to seduce her to get back at her. I wasn't sure, but I did know that eventually I would have to forgive her.

* * *

When school started again, I began commuting from the house in Danville and found that I liked my new lifestyle. At the fraternity, we were up late every night and trying to get out of bed for an eight o'clock class seemed so difficult. But living on my own seemed so much healthier. I could get up earlier and I could go to bed when I wanted to.

I found myself thinking about JoAnn a lot. She had been my first love. We had dated during my senior year in high school and for about half of my freshman year at Cal. Now that I wasn't caught up in the Greek social scene, I found myself thinking about her and realized that she was the only girl I had ever truly loved. But we had broken up because of the social pressures of being a freshman in the Greek system and feeling like you were suppose to go to parties with sorority girls. I had allowed peer pressure to supersede my own instincts. How silly it all sounded now.

I also remembered how caring and loving JoAnn was. She had been through a lot in her own life. I began feeling as if JoAnn and I had more in common than I ever realized. My life had always been so easy, but now I'd had to face some adversity too.

I remembered how attracted I was to both her beauty and her loving personality. I had thrown it all away because I wanted to experience college and the Greek system. I decided that I wanted to see her again.

For her birthday on October 23, I bought her a blank card with a red rose on the cover and wrote a note wishing her a happy birthday. I didn't leave my phone number. She knew I was a member of the Zete House and I figured that if she wanted to contact me, she could.

I didn't hear from her, though I hadn't expected to. I called her mother's house about ten days later. Her stepmother remembered me and was happy to give me her number.

I called JoAnn and we talked the way we always had. I called her again a week or so later. That time, I told her all about my cancer and what it had done to my face. As I would have guessed, JoAnn put a positive spin on it. She reminded me that I was lucky to be alive and that she was sure I didn't look as bad as I thought. I asked if she wanted to get together.

"I'd love to," she said.

We planned to get together for dinner. She lived about fifteen minutes away from where I was living, so we decided to have dinner locally.

I knocked on the door of the house she was renting with her roommates. She opened the door, displaying the smile I missed so much. She barely looked at my face.

"Hi," she said.

"Hey, JoAnn. It's good to see you."

"It's great to see you."

We hugged. She felt great. She looked great, and I knew right away that I wanted to rekindle our relationship.

There was no tension at dinner. We talked as if we had only been apart for a weekend. After dinner we had a drink. Then I offered to take her home. It was late, probably close to midnight.

"I don't want to go home. My roommates are all home."

"Well, where do you want to go?" I asked, letting her set the agenda for the rest of the evening.

"Wherever you want to go."

"Do you want to check out the house I'm living at?"

"Yeah. That sounds good."

I couldn't believe what was happening. She wanted to spend more time with me, and she wanted me to take her to my place. Tyler was gone that night and had told me he wouldn't be home. I was psyched.

I showed JoAnn around a little. She seemed more interested in talking. We talked until about 2:00 in the morning. She was sitting on my bed. I was standing next to the stereo, about ten feet away.

There was a moment of silence. We looked into each other's eyes.

"Can I kiss you?" I asked her. My heart began to pound faster and faster.

"Yes."

JoAnn and I kissed and touched for a while. Then we made love. She was beautiful. I told her I loved her. She told me she loved me. It was happening so fast. But for some reason it didn't seem to be happening fast at all. We knew each other. We had dated before. Though it had been four years ago, it seemed like yesterday.

When I awoke the next morning, JoAnn was asleep next to me. I got up from bed and went outside to grab the newspaper. When I got back, JoAnn was putting on her clothes. We both felt somewhat embarrassed about what had happened and about the way we looked at that moment. Then I offered to take her home. Though I wanted to spend more time with her, I didn't want to push her. I wanted to give her her space.

When we got back to her house, we stepped out of the car and talked a little more. I told her I would call her later. As I drove away, I thanked God that there were people like JoAnn in the world. She seemed to care for me the way she had before. It didn't seem to matter what I looked like. She was so sweet, like an angel sent down to heal my mental wounds.

JoAnn and I continued to date for another six weeks. We enjoyed each other—but what I didn't know that first night was that she had just broken up with a long-term boyfriend. He wanted to get back together with her, and she still loved him.

I kept giving her grief about why she was spending time with me, questioning whether she even liked me at all or whether she just went out with me because she felt sorry for me. I couldn't accept that maybe she did like me for who I was. I drove her away. I drove her back toward her old boyfriend. Whether she

liked me or not, I just wasn't going to believe it. I didn't know
how to just accept things the way they were. I assumed she had a
hidden agenda. I needed a lot of reassurance from her that I was
really an okay, normal guy. I realized after we broke up that I
had a long, long way to go to get my confidence and self-esteem
back.

*   *   *

I continued my routine of school, work and exercise in the
spring semester. I occasionally stopped by the Newman Center
to thank God for my survival and to pray that my cancer wouldn't
recur. I prayed that my reconstruction would be successful, whenever God chose to complete it. I prayed that I would regain my
confidence.

I visualized that my cancer had been washed clean of my
body. I even visualized how I would look when the reconstruction on my face was complete. I imagined that each procedure
that lay ahead of me would bring me closer and closer to Terry.

By the end of the semester I was able to have some more
surgery. A reconstructive eye surgeon tried—unsuccessfully—
to lift my eye with more cartilage from my ears, and Cravens
made some more modifications. Once again, the procedures were
largely successful to the doctors, but barely noticeable to the
layperson. To me, they were frustrating.

I moved back to my parents' for my last semester at Cal in
the Fall of 1987. Because I was planning to have some more
surgery, I didn't think it made a lot of sense to rent an apartment
or a house with anyone.

Cravens finally suggested stepping down as my plastic surgeon. He knew I wanted more done to my face and realized that
my expectations were beyond the scope of his reconstructive
expertise. After all, he was first and foremost an oncologist.

He suggested that I go see a doctor in Chicago by the name
of Ronald Brighton. Cravens didn't know how much money or

time I would be willing to invest in my reconstruction, but he told me that he thought Brighton was the best nasal reconstructive surgeon in the United States. Because one of my best fraternity friends was attending Northwestern's business school in Evanston at the time, I planned to fly out to see him and meet with Brighton at the same time. The timing worked out great. I went to see Brighton a couple of months before graduation, and we agreed that I could begin reconstruction six months later, in January 1988.

Brighton was different from any of the other doctors I'd met. I expected a typical, busy doctor who would spend fifteen minutes at most in the initial consultation. But Brighton spent over three hours discussing my options for reconstruction. He showed me picture after picture of similar defects and their reconstructive outcomes. His work was amazing. He was careful to tell me that the pictures and the portfolio he was showing me were his greatest success stories. He was clear that there could be no guarantees, but he also wanted me to see the stupendous possibilities.

Because of the time Brighton gave me during that initial consultation, I knew that he either truly loved and believed in his work, or saw my case as a great challenge and opportunity. Either way, I was sold. I couldn't wait to begin the reconstruction. The flights back and forth to Chicago would be expensive, but while I was there I would be in the hospital. I figured that I could cover the costs of the flights and other incidentals with the money I had been saving.

My parents supported me one hundred percent. If I believed in Brighton, they would support me emotionally and financially. My mother insisted on going with me, as she felt that I would need the support.

Brighton agreed with Cravens that the best approach was to use a full-thickness skin graft of tissue from my forehead to provide the tissue needed for my columella and right ala. He also planned to use rib cartilage to help define my nostril and bring some symmetry back to my face.

The flap, or "pedicle," would be cut from the upper part of my forehead. That tissue, about the size of a quarter, would be stretched down to my nose, where it would dangle for three weeks to insure that the tissue had developed a new blood supply. Then I would return for more surgery to remove the pedicle and re-shape my nose.

Brighton warned me that I would have to take a few steps backward in order to ultimately go forward and see positive results. I was initially shocked at the prospects of going backward, or having to look worse before looking any better. I didn't realize at the time that I could look that much worse. The brutal truth was that all the reconstruction Dr. Cravens had performed would more or less go to waste. All the tissue transplanted from my chest would be eliminated and replaced by tissue from my forehead.

I thought about my chest and shoulder scars. It looked like a bear had clawed at my chest. All that work was for naught, though the scars on my chest continued to be a source of insecurity whenever I took my shirt off in public. Taking my shirt off at the beach or on the basketball court became a frightening experience in itself. The stares and the questions were as common as those about my face.

The transplant of forehead tissue apparently had a higher success rate to reconstruct noses than did the chest flap. Technology and science were moving at a fast pace. Forehead tissue transplants apparently were unheard of only a few years prior. The skin coloration from my forehead would match my nose and cheek better and the pliability of the forehead tissue was considered superior to that of chest tissue. I also was informed that scarring would be minimal from the forehead donor site. Though all three layers of tissue would be removed from my forehead, the scar tissue that filled the cavity tended to look pretty tame and unnoticeable on many of the patients in Dr. Brighton's portfolio.

Had I made a mistake in not consulting other plastic surgeons a long time ago? I dismissed my musings and decided I had to forget about the past and just plan for my future.

* * *

I was getting excited about my prospects and about life again. Graduating from Cal was an accomplishment. But when I saw the graduation photos of myself, I wished no photographs had been taken of the event. I looked like a monster. I threw away the pictures. My memories of receiving my diploma were clouded by how repulsive I thought I looked on the stage. I wanted to forget the last few years and just look ahead. Things had to get better.

I had to mentally prepare myself for what lay ahead. Dr. Brighton estimated that it could take anywhere from four to six months to complete the reconstruction of my nose, cheek and upper lip. Dr. Brighton recommended doing the procedures at approximately six-week intervals. Though only allowing six weeks between procedures was aggressive, Dr. Brighton also knew how anxious I was to get all this behind me. The original estimate was that I would need to have about four procedures to reconstruct me back to a satisfactory status. Dr. Brighton made it clear that I could take this as far as I chose, but he felt that he could achieve a pretty positive result within four procedures.

* * *

January 8 was my first date of surgery in Chicago. I checked into the hospital the night before so that I could have the lab work done and all the other usual procedures. I met with Dr. Brighton late the night before surgery. He was as chipper as if it were 9:00 a.m.. It didn't seem unusual for him to be working late. I gathered quickly that he worked even longer hours than Dr. Cravens.

As Dr. Brighton looked me over, he decided that it would probably be better to alter his original procedural plan. On further review of my face, he determined that it would make more sense to open up the nose and prepare it with more support tissue before excising the flap and building new tissue around my nose. Though he was going to improve the appearance of my upper lip with a cheek flap and re-cut the scars on my chest, the nose was going to be a little more complicated than he had at first thought.

Why didn't any of this surprise me anymore? The reconstruction of my nose was not clear-cut. Dr. Brighton wanted to get inside of my nose and look around before transplanting any new tissue to the area.

As it turned out, I awoke in the recovery room to find I had bandages and sutures in my groin area, on my chest, on my ears and on my face. For the first time, I was going to leave the hospital with bandages covering my face. Dr. Brighton had opened up my nostril and the result was an extremely unflattering view of the insides of my nose.

I had decided to take a leave of absence from the law firm, until I was satisfied I could dedicate myself 100% to holding a job. I didn't think it was fair for them to employ me when I was planning to be off for two to three weeks, on for two or three weeks and then off again. Fortunately, the law firm was giving me an open invitation to return to work whenever I was ready.

Though Dr. Brighton was able more or less to maintain the aggressive six week interval schedule with me, I quickly discovered that the four-procedure estimate was now going to be more like a five or six-procedure process. Though I was disappointed, I wasn't going to give up. I still had confidence in my doctor and I still was 100% committed to going through the reconstruction, whatever it took.

*　　*　　*

It wasn't until June 2nd that the forehead flap procedure was performed. Dr. Brighton had removed a lot of rib cartilage to build up my inner nostril, ala and columella. My ears had been pretty raped of remaining cartilage. Dr. Brighton assured me that there would be no shortage of cartilage as long as he continued to borrow it from my ribs. Because stripping rib cartilage can be so painful to the patient, Dr. Brighton had gone so far as to store a big chunk of cartilage below my rib cage, just under the skin. That way, he could borrow in the future as needed, and I would incur no real pain, just a few sutures.

*   *   *

It seemed that wearing bandages during this reconstructive phase had suddenly become the norm for me. I tried to socialize as much as I felt comfortable socializing. Originally, I felt more confident with the bandages because I anticipated little reaction from people. My scars and my deformity were covered up. But I found that the bandages in some ways drew more attention to me. People were now more inclined to ask questions than ever before. Because they couldn't see the defect, they were less sensitive and less considerate. I hypothesized that when you have a defect that someone can see, one that appears permanent, people are far more embarrassed to ask questions.

One Friday night my brother Brian and I decided to go have dinner at Pinky's Pizza in Walnut Creek.

Though I had a great big bandage taped over my nose, I had gotten somewhat dressed up. I was wearing jeans but had a starched, yellow button-down shirt on. The pizza was going to take about thirty minutes to prepare. I sat back down at the bar with Brian and started drinking my beer out of a nice cold mug.

I was seated to Brian's right and my bandage was of course covering part of the right side of my face. To my right, I noticed an older gentleman turning his head to look at me over and over again. I finally turned to him to see if he was going to address me or if he was just trying to stare at me without my noticing. He was ready and waiting for me.

"Hey, what in the hell happened to you, partner? Did ya run into a door jam or something?" he half-slurred, laughing hysterically to his buddy next to him.

He was probably in his fifties, had a big beer belly and looked like he had been a shit kicker in his day. He was half drunk. My instinct was to say, "None of your fucking business!" but instead I decided I'd play a little game with him.

I looked him in the eye. "You wanna know the truth?" I asked.

"The truth'd be nice," he replied, laughing again to his partner.

"Well," I said. "Do you have a few minutes?"

"I got all the time in the world," he said.

"Well, it happened like this," I said. I proceeded to tell the guy that I had been hired out of college as a special agent for the DEA. I told him that after close to a year as an agent I had been assigned to work with the Border Patrol in Texas to try to stop some of the marijuana drug-runners that were crossing the border. I described to him the terrain that made it somewhat difficult to monitor and surveil the drug runners. I told him that I was on surveillance with some Border Patrol Agents, viewing the scene from an American suburban vehicle. I was in the passenger seat. It was dusk. Out of nowhere I heard gunfire. Before I had a chance to prepare and cover myself, a shot rang out and pierced through my window, ripping through my cheek and nose.

"No shit?" he remarked, his jaw wide open. He turned to his buddy. "Hey, this guy's a DEA agent. Got shot."

Suddenly I was a hero to this guy. I felt a little guilty, but it was too late to change my story.

"Hey, bartender. Get me another pitcher for my new friend and his buddy," the drunk said.

Brian kicked me under my stool, obviously getting a real laugh out of the whole thing. I knew if I turned to Brian I would start laughing and lose total credibility with this guy.

I continued my story. I told him that after I had been shot I resigned from the agency. Now I was undergoing reconstruction to fix up my nose.

The guy bought it hook, line and sinker. I was feeling even worse because I was making the DEA look like a bunch of unprepared fools, which I knew they were not. But then I thought about it and realized I had told the guy what he wanted to hear. He wouldn't have been comfortable talking about cancer. It would have been too heavy for him. Then I realized I had once again passed judgment on someone on only a few words and an appearance.

"I admire you for your courage," he said. "You're a true American. Sons a bitches who shot you. Shit, you were trying to protect our country and look what happened. Young college kid like you trying to do good. I admire you son."

"Good luck to you, partner," he said.

"Take care," I said, never smiling, playing the part of a real hard ass who takes a bullet like a man.

Brian and I laughed after they had gone out the door. Brian was impressed that I had maintained for as long as I had. The drunk was probably going to tell all his buddies about me.

*   *   *

Though I had to wait six weeks before the forehead flap could be excised, I was fortunate to be able to leave the hospital only a few days after the procedure. What made it bearable was that a big bandage covered the whole flap very nicely. Yes, it was a large bandage, but at least I could cover the deformity and the flap and go out into the real world.

One of my fraternity brothers had invited me to his wedding in Pebble Beach that summer. At the reception, I ran into Peter, my former alumni advisor to the fraternity.

Peter had been very supportive of me after my diagnosis. He had sent me cards in the hospital and had tried to help me deal with some of my social fears after my disfigurement. He was not shy. He was able to ask personal questions without being nosy. He truly liked people and wanted to learn about people's triumphs and tragedies.

I had opened up to him a little when I saw him at Cal football games after I had had my cancer surgery. I had told him I was having self-esteem problems and was lacking in confidence. I didn't open up to just anyone, but Peter had a way of getting things out of me.

As soon as he began speaking, he turned the focus on me and how I was doing with my reconstruction. Putting a positive spin on things, I told him things were going well and that I was going to have a couple more reconstructive procedures done and then would probably start looking for a job.

He asked what I was interested in from a career standpoint. At that time my interests were in working for the DEA or even some insurance company in a claims investigator capacity to try to get some investigative experience. I wanted to eventually go back to law school.

"Why don't you come work for me?" he asked.

Knowing he worked for a computer company and clearly aware of my inexperience with computers except for a class I took for six weeks and then dropped, I told him the truth, which was that I knew nothing about computers. What I didn't tell him was that I wasn't really interested in the computer industry either.

"It doesn't matter that you don't know anything about computers now. Believe me, you'll learn very quickly. I think you'd be great in sales or anything else for that matter."

I was flattered that Peter wanted to talk to me about a job. What was more flattering was that he was talking about me being hired in a sales capacity. I had been wondering whether I could ever sell, given my deformity. I didn't know if I would be given an opportunity and I wasn't sure I was ready to get in front of groups of people.

"Why don't you call me Monday morning?" he suggested. "I get in before 7:00 every morning. Call me and we'll set up an appointment."

I couldn't say no. He hadn't offered me a job yet. But what really made me feel good was that he was willing to talk to me about a job knowing I had cancer and facial disfigurement. He worked for a small company and I knew a thing or two about pre-existing conditions already. My father had warned me that getting insurance might be difficult and that I would probably be better off working for a larger company that was in a better position to insure me.

I left the reception feeling a little better about myself, knowing that Peter must have seen some qualities in me that would warrant him setting up an appointment with me for a possible job.

*   *   *

Peter's company, Granite Computer Products, Inc., was riding the Personal Computer distribution wave and had grown from $4 million in sales its first year (1986) to $8 million the next. The 1988 projection was $16 million. Fortunately for me, he had an immediate need for someone to manage the customer service department. It was an opportunity to build a process and develop procedures and guidelines and methods for tracking service issues, product repairs, returns and credits. The company was growing so fast that within six months there would be an opportunity for me either in inventory management (purchasing) or sales.

Peter offered me the job and asked me when I could start. I asked for a couple of days to think about it. When I talked with my dad about it, he expressed concern about medical insurance but otherwise told me it was a decision I had to make for myself.

The next day, I called Peter and told him I was excited about the opportunity but had concerns about medical coverage, given that I had a pre-existing condition. He assured me that wouldn't be a problem. I told him that I would prefer to keep my existing coverage under COBRA and asked if Granite would cover the monthly fee of close to $200.

"Absolutely. All you need to do is submit an expense report each month and I'll approve it."

I also told him I would prefer to start after I had recovered from my next procedure, which was scheduled for a month later.

"I have the spot open for you whenever you want to take it," he said. "Just keep in touch."

I accepted the job.

CHAPTER FIFTEEN

New Challenges

Brighton had scheduled my next procedure on August 8. Things were coming together. The tissue and cartilage were taking, and the coloration of the new skin matched that of the existing tissue. The doctor planned to make a few more improvements but warned me that I might need additional surgery down the road.

So much had been done over the past seven months that he wanted to take some time out and let the healing process run its course. He was afraid of tweaking what he had already reconstructed. I still had a tremendous amount of swelling, and some of what he had done might have started to pull toward the cavity in my right maxillary area under all the new cartilage and tissue he had transplanted. Only time would tell.

I was tired of hospitals and surgery, tired of recovering, tired of battling to get back into physical shape and then have to lay off while things healed. I wanted to have a new purpose and one that I could control. I was ready to start a career. I had the rest of my life to fix my face. For the first time since my major cancer surgery, reconstruction wasn't my number one priority.

I was surprised to find myself feeling that way, but a lot of that feeling was coming from the fact that my progress was slow, and not as successful as I had hoped. I had had a lot of reconstruction and so much of it had required that I take steps backwards in order to make future steps forward. I had come to realize finally that reconstructing my face might be a little more than a short-term project. I would have to learn patience above all else. I would wait to hear back from the doctor before I pushed for any more surgery. I would stay in touch with Dr. Brighton, but when he felt the time would be right, I would be ready. It was time for a break, for all of us. Besides, the idea of starting a career had me excited, and I needed to be excited about something.

The true reality was beginning to sink in. Though Brighton had made tremendous improvements to my face and nose, I still was a long way from being the old Terry. How much more could I take, really? I had been through three times the number of procedures I had expected to go through already. Why not work for awhile and see how things went.

I was fortunate that my family could help support me financially and emotionally. The time had come though to live my own life the way God had intended for me to live it.

Brighton hadn't given up yet, but my case was difficult, involving the loss of muscle, bone and cartilage and affecting my eye, nose, cheek, and lip. Most patients needed reconstruction for only their nose or only their lip. I realized that none of the patients I'd seen in Brighton's portfolio had started out with as much damage as I had.

*　　*　　*

After the August 8 procedure, my face showed marked improvement but was still far from symmetrical. With the forehead flap removed, Dr. Brighton was able to create a more normal-looking nostril and ala on my right side. The nostril wasn't functional and never would be, but after almost three years of living without one on that side, I had gotten used to the feeling of breathing through one side of my nose. I wasn't willing to endure another set of procedures just to regain the functionality of that nostril.

Also, my nose was finally straight again. The scar line along the bridge of my nose was hardly noticeable and my cheek skin coloration looked better. But now I had a scar that ran from my right eyebrow all the way up my forehead. The quarter-size donor site on my forehead still hadn't totally healed. Dr. Brighton had fixed my upper lip, but in so doing had created a zigzag scar from my upper chin all the way along the right side of my lip. Part of that reconstruction had also pulled the right side of my upper lip upwards, thinning the lip on the right side and elevating it so that my teeth were sometimes visible even when I wasn't smiling.

I knew I looked a lot better, but I also had some brand-new scars that would take years to heal. Brighton thought my forehead scar would all but disappear within a couple of years but as it turned out, it and the other scars became very red and have never really faded away.

When I left Chicago without scheduling any more reconstructive procedures, I really wanted to think about something besides my face. I didn't know then that my next trip back to Brighton would lead to one of the happiest episodes in my life since I had been diagnosed with cancer. But that happiness would also uncover a new obstacle, in many ways more challenging than any I had confronted yet.

*   *   *

I began my job on August 30, 1988, and immersed myself in work. I got into the office at 6:30 a.m. daily for product training and at 7:00 a.m. I began working, trying to catch up on the previous night's work before the phones started ringing at 8:00. I worked until 7:00 p.m. most nights. The job was the perfect way for me to forget about my personal problems. I loved the company. I loved my job. I loved the challenge that I had been given. I was on my own.

The problem was that I began to use the job as a shield against the outside world. It became my excuse. I couldn't go out with friends because I had to work. I made time for my exercise program, but beyond that I made little time for anything else. I wasn't meeting any new girls. I felt better about myself, but not great. The reconstruction had given me a little more confidence, but I still shied away from going to parties or bars. I still felt as if I would be noticed wherever I went. Time would heal me, I told myself. The busier I was, the faster time would go by.

But sometimes I wondered how I could have gone from being so confident in myself that I always kept my head up, looking out for pretty girls—to now being so insecure that I kept my head down wherever I went, fearing that some pretty girl might be looking at me out of curiosity rather than out of desire.

I was still under medical care for my condition at UCSF. I had CT scans regularly, but was told that after two years with no recurrence I would only need to have the CT scan once a year. After five years, I would be considered cured.

I drove out to UCSF myself for my next CT scan. Afterwards, I planned to stop by Fourteen Long and Eleven Long to say hello to the nurses that had been so instrumental in my care. I couldn't believe that more than two years had gone by since my care there. I had lost touch with all the nurses. I had spoken to them a couple of times on the telephone, but not recently. I had been interested in Carolyn and Claire, but feared I'd be rejected if I tried to get dates with them. I felt that if I saw them now, enough time would have passed that it would be clear I wasn't here for a date. And I wasn't, though I wouldn't have said no if one of them had asked me out.

After six surgeries in Chicago, I realized the difference in the care they had given me. UCSF nurses were worlds ahead of the nursing care I received in Chicago. They were more professional and they were a hell of a lot cuter.

* * *

As I approached the nurse's station on Fourteen Long, I recognized no one.

"Hi," I said. "I was wondering if I could say a quick hello to a few of the nurses that cared for me here a couple of years ago."

"Sure," one of the nurses replied. "Who are you looking to see?"

"Carolyn, Kathleen or Adrienne," I said, hopefully.

"Let's see. I'm trying to think. Carolyn Clary, right?"

"Ya, that's it," I said, realizing Carolyn was the only one who's last name I knew.

Carolyn had moved to the emergency room, Kathleen was teaching, Adrienne was working in the recovery room and when I got to the eleventh floor, I found out Claire had gotten married and moved to San Diego.

I couldn't believe that not one of them was still there, but as I thought about it, it did not surprise me. It would probably be very difficult to care for cancer patients for a long period of time. Seeing patients die frequently would probably wear on anyone very quickly. It occurred to me that none of my favorite nurses were in the kind of capacity now that would even allow for visitors.

* * *

Everyone had moved on with their lives. They all had brand-new lives, and I had to make a new life for myself as well. I had to move on from the safe haven of the hospital and my cancer treatment and reconstruction.

I left the hospital. A lot can happen in two years, I thought to myself. I hoped my life might change over the coming two years.

*　　*　　*

A couple of weeks later, I asked my brother Rob if he would be interested in going to the Catholic Church near UCSF with me on some Sunday to attend Mass. I had found out that the 'Take it Away' guy was a lector there, and I wanted to find him and thank him for the power of his prayers. This time, my healer was there for me to thank. Though I didn't know this man like I knew my nurses, his two minutes in my room had affected me as much as my nurses' gifts over the weeks they had cared for me.

He spoke with such passion and compassion that the people in the church listened with rapt admiration. He didn't just read like so many lectors do. After Mass, I made a dash for the exit. He was already talking to a group of women. I looked away briefly, and when I turned back, he was gone.

"Shit, Rob, where is he?"

"He was just there a second ago," Rob replied. He had missed him step away also.

I started running down the street and saw him walking so briskly up the hill toward the hospital that he was almost running. I started running after him. By the time I approached him, he had stopped to talk to a couple he apparently knew.

As he said good-bye to them, I stepped forward. "Excuse me," I said. "You probably don't remember me, but you gave me the host at UC a couple of years ago after I'd had cancer surgery."

"Yes." He looked at me blankly.

"I just wanted to thank you for your passionate prayer. You don't know how much of an impact it had on me. I can still remember it clearly today."

"Good. I'm glad." He didn't smile.

"You have a real gift. I just wanted you to know that I am healthy and my cancer is gone."

"Good. I'm happy for you. If you'll excuse me, I'm late for an appointment."

"No problem. Thank you," I said.

I watched him leave and thought that his satisfaction was not in being thanked for what he had done, but for doing what he loved to do. I was happy that I had tracked him down. He did exist. He was a human being. He was not Jesus Christ, as I had occasionally wondered over the past couple of years.

*   *   *

A year passed in the blink of an eye. I sent Brighton Polaroid shots of my face every few months so that he could see the changes in my face. My nose had started to turn toward the right, toward the cavity in my maxillary area. He thought he could straighten out my nose, among other things. He also felt like enough time had passed that we could move forward with the next procedure.

We scheduled the surgery for September 19, 1989. Besides straightening out the nose, he planned to fix some of the scarring on my forehead. The removal of tissue had caused a slant in my right eyebrow that had become very noticeable. The eyebrow itself appeared higher than the other side due to the contraction toward the donor site scar on the upper part of my forehead. Brighton also wanted to reshape my right nostril a little by grafting more rib cartilage into my nose and to open the airway slightly. He also planned to "de-fat" my upper lip cheek graft so that it would not protrude above the adjacent tissue.

The surgery was substantial. There were definite improvements. Although he used some of my rib cartilage to reshape my nose, a big chunk of cartilage was left sitting in a lump under the right side of my rib cage. I wondered if I would ever get rid of that ball of hard matter. But that was really the least of my concerns. What was one more bump and one more scar?

For the first time since seeing Dr. Brighton, I had gone to Chicago alone. I probably would never have met Dina, the attractive girl down the hall from me, if my mother had been there.

*   *   *

I was feeling pretty good the day after my surgery. I was told I could walk up and down the hallways as much as I felt like it. Somewhat bored, I found myself walking up and down the same hallways about once every two hours, shuffling up and down the corridors and glancing into the patient rooms to see whom I was sharing the floor with. Most of the patients were elderly. I noticed that in one room there was a patient that always seemed to have visitors crowding over her. The first couple of times I glanced in the room I saw an older woman and a couple of young girls laughing and carrying on. They looked like fun people, people I might want to meet. I decided to make my walks even more frequent in hopes I could get a look inside at whoever was in that bed. I knew it was a girl, because I had heard her voice. Her voice was sexy, but I wanted to know what she looked like too.

I was a hypocrite. Why did I have to get a look at her to decide whether or not I would be interested in meeting her? Why was I still so judgmental? As I passed her room again, I noticed that her two visitors had moved to the far side of her bed, away from the door. I kept on walking, pretending I wasn't fazed by whatever was going on inside that room.

The girl in the bed was gorgeous—shoulder-length dark-brown hair, thick eyebrows, clear skin, and seductive eyes that locked onto mine for that brief millisecond that was enough for me to make a point to meet her as soon as possible. For all I knew, she might check out of the hospital that day.

The next time my nurse Susan checked on me, I asked her if she wouldn't mind doing me a big favor.

In the most appreciative manner I could muster I asked her, "Would you mind doing a little research for me?"

"Sure. What do you need?" she grinned.

"Find out who is in room 802A. The girl in the bed closest to the window looks really cute."

Susan laughed and walked off giggling. "Sure." It was probably the first time she had ever been involved in matchmaking for her patients.

What was I thinking? I had bandages in two places on my face. One bandage stretched across the upper part of my nose and eyebrow and the other stretched over my upper lip and cheek area. I looked as if a truck had just hit me. But for some reason I was more confident, partly because bandages and swelling were acceptable in a hospital environment. Besides, at least my hair had been cleaned and combed that day.

A couple of hours later, Susan appeared at my door and motioned me into the hallway.

"I'd like you to meet a friend of mine," she said as I approached her in my robe and slippers. "Come on."

I followed her down the hall, knowing exactly where she was taking me but realizing that Susan was only going to make the introductions and leave it at that. Dina and I totally hit it off. She was easy to talk to. She was full of energy, something I had always found very attractive.

I opened myself up to Dina in no time at all. After only five minutes of 'get-acquainted' talk, I told her directly why I had asked my nurse to introduce us. I told Dina I felt I had nothing to lose by asking to meet her. If I didn't introduce myself, I told her, the chances were good that I might never see her again. I told her that I found her very attractive and was determined to meet her.

Surprisingly, her response was immediate and serious. "I felt the same way about you. I was talking to my friends about meeting you. Every time you walked by my mom would say, 'there goes the guy in the white robe.' My girlfriend told me I should meet you. But I'm stuck in this bed at least until tomorrow. I can't even get out of bed. So there wasn't much I could do about it."

We openly told each other what we found attractive about one another. I told her she had a classic look and beautiful eyes and skin. She told me she had seen me walking by from a distance but had still been attracted to me right off the bat.

Dina was in the hospital because of a blood clot in her leg. She had been out to dinner with her mother and two girlfriends when she collapsed from the pain in her leg as she tried to stand up. She was going to be fine, but her leg was wrapped and she had to stay in bed for several days to insure that the clot subsided. I described my cancer and the reconstruction that I was going through.

She peered at me and said she liked my high cheekbone on the left side of my face. She said that that the right cheekbone was collapsed 'a little bit' but wasn't that noticeable.

My nose was visible. My eyes were visible. The bandage only covered some sutured areas on my eyebrow and upper lip. I was shocked by her comments. I had never even thought of my cheekbones as the most noticeable defect. I had always felt most self-conscious about my nose and eye.

"You're a really good-looking guy. All you should really do is have your cheekbone fixed—if you really want to. But it's not a big deal."

Had God sent this girl down from heaven? She had delivered the biggest shot in the arm I had received in years. I wondered why she was saying the things she said. Why would anyone tell me, unsolicited, that I was good-looking? Maybe I wasn't as bad off as I thought. Maybe my ugliness was only in my own head.

"I should leave you alone," I said. "I just wanted to introduce myself." I have to admit that I was testing her to see if she was really interested.

"No. Don't leave. Let's keep talking."

*   *   *

We talked some more. We learned more about each other and found that our backgrounds were somewhat similar. She was a little younger, but had just graduated from Northwestern University, and was pursuing a career in television broadcasting as a news reporter.

I went back to my room for dinner. An hour or so later the telephone rang.

"Hello," I said.

"Hi. It's Dina. Why don't you come down for a while."

"I'll be right there."

I jumped out of bed and ran to the bathroom. I looked at myself. Though I wasn't happy with what I saw, I decided it wasn't worth fixing myself up. There wasn't much I could do to look any better.

As I rounded the corner into her room, I noticed a guy standing next to her with flowers and some snacks. I stopped at the door, hesitating to enter. It occurred to me that her visitor was probably her boyfriend. I had to be a big boy about it. I couldn't turn away.

"Come on in," Dina said. "This is Jeff. Jeff, this is Terry. Jeff is a friend of mine from Northwestern. Terry is a patient here, obviously."

Jeff didn't smile. Dina opened the snacks and began sharing them with Jeff and me. She made it clear that Jeff was just a friend. After he left, about fifteen minutes later, she told me that he had been after her for a while but that she wasn't interested in him.

*   *   *

My cousin Megan had been living in Chicago at that time and had brought Chinese food to share with me one afternoon. Eating food from the outside world was a real treat, but I still ate everything they served me at the hospital because I knew my body needed the nutrients. Besides, food was food as far as I was concerned, and the hospital food wasn't that bad. Dina, on the other hand, hated hospital food. She told me that she hadn't eaten her dinner that night.

The next day I remembered the leftover Chinese food. Around lunchtime, I asked my nurse if she could retrieve it from the refrigerator for me. Minutes later, I strolled into Dina's room with two plates of microwave heated Chinese food.

"Oh, you're awesome. This looks great!" she shouted.

Dina gobbled down her share of the leftover chow mein, broccoli and beef and steamed rice. When we finished eating, Dina pulled out a bottle of Chardonnay that a friend had given her.

"What do you say we pop this tonight after dinner?"

"Sounds good to me."

Dina was a ball of energy. I was starting to think she liked me.

We got back together after dinner. Dina had been given permission to walk that day. We strolled down to the waiting room down the hall and opened our wine. I had taken a couple of glasses from our serving trays before they were picked up so that we would have something to drink out of. Dina's friend had given her a corkscrew. We drank wine and talked until 2:00 a.m..

As we sipped our wine, I offered to take Dina to the Napa Valley wine country if she ever came out to California. She accepted and told me she wouldn't forget. I wasn't so sure.

The next morning after breakfast I stepped into my bathroom to get cleaned up. When I opened my door to return to my bed, I saw Dina lying in my bed with the sheets up to her waist.

"Hey, Terry. You wanna join me?" she said.

I looked over at my roommate. He was somewhat out of it, probably in shock.

"She's just a friend," I said. "I hope it doesn't offend you."

He just looked at me and shook his head. I was a little embarrassed. What would the nurses think? How comfortable was my roommate with all this, really? I wondered. I guess I didn't care that much.

I was a little hesitant to join Dina in the bed, so I leaned against the windowsill.

We talked most of the morning. Both of us were scheduled

for release at noon that day. I had my sutures removed. I showered and dressed. Dina did the same.

Dina's boss arrived to pick her up a little before I planned to leave. Dina called me over to her room and we agreed to stay in touch. She kissed my cheek and gave me a big hug. I held her for a long time. I hoped I'd see her again but thought I probably wouldn't.

*   *   *

On the plane trip home all I thought about was Dina. I'd had more fun in the hospital during those few days than I'd had anywhere else in a long time. I felt as if God had been watching over me. The next day about noon, the phone rang.

"Hi, Terry. This is Dina. Is your offer still good?"

"Absolutely."

That first month, before she came out, my phone bill to Dina alone was $168.00. We talked for at least three hours almost every night.

Dina ended up coming out for three nights. We spent the first night at my parents' house, and they fell in love with her just as I'd expected. We spent the second night in San Francisco and the third in the Napa Valley. We enjoyed each other, we made love many times, we laughed a lot. The last night, we got into a fight.

I hadn't realized it, but I had worn on her a bit. She felt as if she had to constantly tell me how much she liked me. I couldn't believe that she truly liked me, even though she had flown out from Chicago to see me and had already spent two nights with me.

For the first time I realized the burden I must have put on people without being aware of it. Dina wasn't one to sugarcoat anything. She was very direct about her feelings, but my insecurity and lack of confidence had doused the flame she had for me. I had spoiled everything. My problem wasn't my appearance. It was my self-esteem. I was finally aware of the severity of my condition. Dina was a pretty, smart and fun person who liked me, my looks, and my personality but couldn't deal with my insecurity.

Our relationship changed after that weekend. We kept on talking on a fairly regular basis and easily made the transition from lovers to friends. She remains a close friend to this day. The impact she had on me was tremendous. She gave me confidence by giving me her love and attention, but she also taught me about my weaknesses.

My real weaknesses were mental and emotional, not physical. Because of Dina, I began to learn where I would need to focus if I were ever going to move forward with my life. Surgery on my physical scars had to take a back seat to fixing my mental and emotional scars. They had disfigured me far more than the physical deformity ever had.

CHAPTER SIXTEEN

A Better Life

After my experience with Dina I began to integrate myself back into the social circles I had been avoiding since my operations and disfigurement. I had to in order to build back my confidence level. Things at work were great. The company continued to grow, and to offer me new opportunities.

Brighton and I continued to talk on the telephone about my progress. He had suggested that perhaps I undergo another forehead flap to add more skin to the right side of my nose.

I wasn't interested in any more flaps. We did agree that due to the discomfort of the tearing and the self-consciousness I was having with my right eye and the fact that the asymmetry of my eyes now seemed my most prominent defect, perhaps it made sense to consider reconstruction of that area now that I had reached a point of acceptance with my nose and upper lip.

Brighton encouraged me to see Dr. Kitamura, a doctor in Los Angeles whom he described as the best eye reconstructive surgeon in the country. I decided it couldn't hurt to meet him, so I arranged to fly to Los Angeles.

Walking into Kitamura's office, I knew I was in the right place. The waiting room was standing room only and as I glanced around the room I noticed several people with severe defects awaiting their appointments. I saw two children who appeared to have facial and cranial birth defects. I realized there were many other people out there hoping to someday appear 'normal.' But as I looked around, it became clear to me that most of the patients were small children who had never known what it was like to look 'normal'. They had been born disfigured. They had probably endured immense pain and loneliness from the criticism and ostracism they encountered from other schoolchildren so prone to dishing out cruel comments to those less fortunate.

Dr. Kitamura had extreme confidence. Well dressed, he was about fifty years of age and appeared to keep himself in good physical condition. He didn't ask a lot of questions. He didn't want to spend a lot of time examining me or selling me on his abilities to repair my eye. In no time, he had a plan to reconstruct my eye.

He suggested transplanting a right temporal muscle flap into my mouth to separate my oral cavity from my nasal cavity. This procedure, though major, would solve several problems. With the oral cavity sealed off, mucous from my upper sinus would no longer drain directly into my mouth. The flap would also fill the cavity in my right cheek and alleviate the pulling of tissue in that direction. Building up my cheek would make my face more symmetrical. Finally, filling the cavity would provide a foundation for the eye; Kitamura would use cranial bone grafts to reconstruct the front part of my cheekbone, which would raise the lower orbit so it would be more in line with my left eye.

The procedure was intended to aid in my hygiene and provide for greater comfort and functionality of my eye and mouth. My upper sinus would finally drain into my nostrils as it was intended to. The pulling sensation I felt from my lower eyelid would hopefully be alleviated as well. The prospect of making my eyes symmetrical again was very encouraging.

On the downside, I was told I would not be able to wear my obturator for two weeks after the procedure. As a result, I had resigned myself to returning to work without six of my upper teeth, including my two front teeth. On top of the appearance insecurity, my speech would also be impaired due to the fact that my palate would be once again altered.

Most of the people at work knew about the reconstruction I was planning. At least I could return to work in a comfortable environment. I wasn't about to ask for two weeks off just because of what my co-workers might have thought when they saw me. I knew I could work, and I could just tell people on the telephone I had had dental work and that was why I was having difficulty with my speech. I planned to postpone all outside meetings, however. I knew that Mark, my boss, would understand. He had been very supportive of giving me time off for reconstruction if I felt it was necessary. As a matter of fact, he had sent me a Sony Walkman and a tape on my last visit to Chicago that consisted of hilarious interviews with people at work. It had left me roaring with laughter.

All in all, Kitamura performed two surgeries on me over a six-month period. Once again, the outcome was successful from a functional standpoint, but within six months my eye had drooped back to its original position.

I wasn't interested in any more reconstruction unless it became necessary for functional reasons. Over the next few years I had several minor procedures performed by various doctors. Several times I developed buildups of scar tissue in my palate and around one of my remaining molars that more than likely had been caused by the transplant of temporal muscle into my mouth. The rapid growth of the scar tissue caused discomfort and resorbtion of the adjacent tooth. I eventually lost count of the number of reconstructive procedures I endured, but it was somewhere near thirty when I last counted.

I finally felt that I didn't need any more reconstruction. I had endured enough and had the experience now to realize that the results would never meet my expectations. Part of the change in attitude was out of my control. Going through reconstruction might make me look worse – there were no guarantees at all. Maybe I wasn't that bad off the way I was. Over time, I learned to accept my fate, remember my experience with Dina, and not forget that my physical appearance was no longer my biggest obstacle to happiness.

I was dating again. I was ready to give something back to those less fortunate. I wanted to help other people. I felt that by sharing my experience I could help and inspire others. I had survived cancer. It had been four years since my radiation. The time had come to move on. So many people had given of themselves to help me. It was my turn to help others in need.

I contacted the Wellness Community, a cancer support organization that provides free group therapy for both cancer patients and their support systems, whether that be friends or family. I felt that by sharing my experience with others I could have a great impact and provide inspiration to those battling not only cancer, but also all the side effects of cancer, such as hair loss, weight loss, and all the other external elements that inhibits our self-esteem and confidence.

I was familiar with the Wellness Community because I had gone there a few years earlier seeking emotional support. I parted from that group at the Wellness Community with a girlfriend, one who also had cancer. In hindsight, I think the reason I attended the group was to try to meet a female who would understand and be sensitive to how cancer and the insecurity associated with it affects our psyche. Though the group was all young adults, the maturity level was higher than one would expect, probably because we were all dealing with adult issues. I had connected myself to the disease in a way I never imagined. I was dating someone with cancer that had just as good a chance of living as dying. I wanted to be there to help her.

The hardest part was realizing that I was dating her for all the wrong reasons. We were not at all alike. She needed more reassurance than I did. Her goal was to find a man she could marry. I wasn't ready for that. We broke up within six weeks.

I realized I didn't need to date someone with cancer to feel like I was helping others with cancer. I didn't have to get that close to it. I could help more people by volunteering at the Wellness Community, not as a therapist, as I was not educated or qualified, but as an Introductory Group Leader. My job was to educate newcomers to the Wellness Community about the different programs available to them. The participants in these groups were generally people who had only recently been diagnosed with cancer. They were facing surgery, chemotherapy and radiation. They were often scared, confused, sad, or even angry.

To qualify to become an Introductory Group Leader one had to have been a cancer victor. I could now say that I was. My doctors had given me a clean bill of health. As one of many leaders for the group, for which I was only responsible once per month, I had to introduce myself, tell them about my cancer experience, and inform them that I was cured. My co-group leader would do the same. We would then ask everyone in the group, whether a patient or a support person, to share their own experiences. Tears were often shed, but by the end of the session most of the participants were charged up and excited about joining a group that could offer support and help in their quest for a richer and fuller life despite the obstacles they were facing.

*   *   *

Interestingly and coincidentally, when I had reached the point in my life where I was ready to try to help others, my brother Rob began his own struggle with a completely different tribulation. He had been combating his own mental, physical, spiritual and emotional challenges for years, but no one in our immediate family had recognized it. Though he had known it since he was twelve years old, it took Rob until he was about thirty to accept the fact that he was gay.

Rob had held his pain inside for so many years, he had managed to mask it from others. When I was diagnosed with cancer, Rob felt that coming out at that point would have been too much for the family to take. He had withheld his true feelings for close to twenty years. Rob told me later that his observance of my struggle with my own emotional, mental, spiritual and physical challenges helped him realize that he could come out. He was about to embark on a journey filled with many of the same struggles I had battled in fitting into a society that doesn't necessarily reward people who are different. The fortunate part for Rob was that our family embraced and accepted him for who he was. Yes, it had been a surprise, but our love for Rob was unconditional, as it had been for me.

*   *   *

One Saturday night in August 1991, shortly after I had broken up with my girlfriend who had cancer, I had attended a cousin's wedding in San Francisco. After the reception ended, around nine o'clock, my brother Brian and I decided to go to Perry's Bar on Union Street. About ten minutes after we arrived, three nicely dressed women walked into the bar. Laughing and seeming to be very upbeat, they quickly grabbed the stools to my left and ordered drinks. Brian and I had almost finished our drinks. We looked at each other. Should we stay or should we go?

"What do you think?" Brian asked. "Do you want to go down the street to another bar or what?"

I thought for a moment. I looked down and to my left at the hands and nicely manicured fingernails of the woman next to me. I listened to her talk for a moment. I quickly shifted in my stool to get a more complete look. She was dressed nicely. She was very pretty. She had that classic look that I always found so attractive.

"How about one more drink? I want to hang out for a minute and see what the deal is with this gal next to me," I told Brian.

Moments later, three older men walked into the bar. Within minutes, they were making moves on the women.

"Hey, this place is a little dead. What do you say we head over to Earl's down the street?" the leader of the pack asked them.

"What's Earl's like?" one of the ladies asked.

Before he could answer, I leaned over to the girl next to me. "You don't want to go to Earl's. Believe me. The average age is about twenty." I was kind of hitting on her, but I was able to hide it pretty well. "It's a new bar over on the corner of Van Ness and Clay, I think."

"Well, where would you suggest we go? We want to go somewhere fun."

"How about Silhouette's in North Beach? They have a dance floor, but it's a little bit of an older crowd."

We introduced ourselves and got to talking. She worked at a travel agency in Palo Alto and had spent the day in Napa with her sister Pam, who was in town from Chicago, and Carolyn, a friend from Boise, Idaho. Sue asked me for my business card. I asked her for hers, but she didn't have one. She told me she worked for a travel agency called Casto Travel.

"It was nice meeting you guys," she said at last. "Have fun tonight. We're heading over to Silhouette's."

After Brian and I finished our drinks, I suggested we head over to Silhouette's too. "This girl's pretty hot," I told him. "Do you mind?"

We grabbed the next cab we could find on Union Street.

We walked into Silhouette's probably twenty minutes behind the girls. The place was packed and I wasn't sure how I was going to approach the girls if I did spot them. Then I saw Sue walking directly toward me from the restroom.

'Oh, no!' I thought to myself 'She's going to think I'm a psycho. She meets me in a bar and then I follow her across town.'

"Hey," she smiled. "How are you guys doing?"

What a relief. She was happy to see me.

"Do you guys want drinks. I'll buy this round," she said.

I was dumbfounded. She was taking the initiative. I knew then I was going to have a fun night.

Brian and I ended up dancing with the three of them until the bar closed. Then Pam invited us back to the Marriott, where the three of them had a room for the night, for another drink and some leftover pizza. Brian and I were starving as usual, and accepted the offer. I was more interested in spending time with Sue. Brian was more interested in eating the pizza.

We ended up hanging out in the room until after 4:00 a.m.. Brian passed out on one of the beds. Pam and Carolyn started signaling that they were ready for bed. I asked Sue if she wanted to get some fresh air.

"Sure," she said.

We walked down the hallway to the elevator. My goal was to go to the top of the hotel and go out on the rooftop for some fresh air and maybe even a view.

Once in the elevator, I asked Sue if I could kiss her. We kissed for a moment and then the elevator door opened. I found an exit door to the roof, but the problem was that it automatically locked when it was closed. I didn't want to get Sue stuck on the roof of the building. We decided to head back to her room. I woke Brian up and we said our good-byes to the girls. I liked Sue a lot, but I didn't know if it was right to pursue her. After all, I had met her in a bar. How many girls did I ever end up dating that I met in bars? Zero.

Brian and I grabbed a cab and got to my brother Steve and his wife Ann's place, where we spent the night. Unbeknownst to me, Brian had discussed meeting the girls at the Chestnut Grill for breakfast later that morning.

I woke up around nine, and a little while later the phone rang. Ann picked it up, listened to the caller, and handed the phone over to Brian.

"It's some girl who said she met you last night?"

"Oh, shit," Brian said. "I didn't give her this number."

"Well, that's weird," Ann said. "Terry, did you give her the number?"

"No," I said. "I gave her one of my cards and told her we were staying at my brother's house in the city. Maybe she called information for Healey and got the number."

"No. She couldn't have gotten the number from information. It's unlisted."

Brian finally went to the back room to talk with Sue. A few minutes later he told me that she wanted to talk to me. I picked up the phone.

"Brian mentioned something about getting together for brunch," Sue said, "so I thought I'd call and make sure we were still on."

"Brunch?" I asked. "I don't know. Brian and I need to head back to Walnut Creek pretty soon."

"Oh, really? Okay, I just wanted to make sure we weren't supposed to meet you. No problem."

"Just out of curiosity, how did you get this number?" I asked.

"Well, you told me you grew up in Walnut Creek. I called information. There was only a couple Healey's spelled H-e-a-l-e-y. Your mom answered and told me you were at Steve and Ann's house in the city. She gave me the number."

I had to admit, I was a little disturbed by her tracking us down. I liked that she was interested, but it seemed extreme to go to all that effort. I was better off sleeping on things for awhile and deciding later if I was still interested. And I couldn't believe my mother. She was a total security breach. She would give any-one a phone number.

There wasn't a whole lot more to say. We both said good-bye.

*   *   *

I thought a lot about Sue the rest of the day. She sure didn't seem like the psycho type, but how would one ever know. I was glad I had cut it off. It just didn't seem right to date a girl I had met in a bar.

I thought more about Sue the rest of the week. She didn't seem like the type who went to bars to meet guys. She was there because she had friends in town and they were staying in the city. I was there because I was at a wedding and decided to just have a couple of drinks. The more I thought about her, the more I realized I didn't care where I had met her. I wanted to see her again but I didn't know her last name or where she lived. Somehow, I had to track her down.

*   *   *

The following Friday night, I had plans to meet a friend in the city. I stopped by the Marriott Hotel. I was dressed professionally and hoped my appearance would help my case with the desk clerk. I needed to hit her up for a big favor.

I walked up to her confidently.

"Hello, sir. How may I help you?" she asked.

"Well, I realize this is an odd request. I know you normally don't give out the names of guests. But I have a problem. I left my briefcase in one of your guests' rooms last Saturday night. One of the girls who was staying in the room called me and left me a message that she had my briefcase. The problem is that my roommate deleted the message and I have no way of contacting her now to get my briefcase back. I know I was on the 33rd floor and I know the first name of the person the room would have been registered under."

I figured that because Sue was a travel agent, she had probably booked the room herself. I knew she was from Palo Alto but I couldn't remember the name of the travel agency she worked for.

"I'm sorry sir. I'm not authorized to give that kind of information out."

I pleaded with her to give me some hint of information that would help in my search. I asked if she could just give me her last name and I would try to figure out the rest.

The clerk—her name was Sheila—told me she would check with her manager and get back to me by phone. I didn't want to push her. I gave her my name and work number and told her that if she left me any messages there, I would be sure my roommate wouldn't erase it. I laughed, hoping to reel her in a little bit, hoping she'd feel sorry for me. It didn't work. She stared at me with a blank face.

* * *

Several days went by. I hadn't heard from Sheila. The following Friday I was in the city again. I again stopped by the Marriott, figuring that the more I could get my face in front of Sheila, the better. I had a suit on. I wanted desperately to make the impression that I was an important and legitimate person.

But Sheila wasn't at the front desk. The clerk on duty told me Sheila was working in billing that night and offered to help me.

I didn't want to start all over. "Actually, it would be easier if you could get her for me."

A few minutes later, Sheila appeared.

I reminded her of my request, but she reiterated the hotel's policy on confidentiality.

"We would be liable if you tracked the guest down and something happened to her. It's not that I don't trust you personally. It's just our policy."

I knew I couldn't keep coming back to the Marriott every week, so I decided to ask to talk with the reservations manager.

A minute or so later, the manager appeared. As soon as he came out to help me, I realized that I might have a good chance of getting what I needed. He was about my age, athletic-looking, and appeared to be the kind of guy who might understand my predicament.

I told him the same story I had told Sheila, except that I told him I was with a girl in the room until about 4:00 a.m., and was so tired when I left that I had forgotten my briefcase. He laughed and asked me to wait for a few minutes.

"Let me see what I can do for you. Do you remember the room number?"

"Well, no. But it was 3335 or 3331 or somewhere around

there. Can you check on a range of numbers close to that for August 3rd?"

"Give me a few minutes."

A short time later, he returned with some reservation slips and began reading off names and home addresses. There was nothing even close to a Sue or an address in Palo Alto.

"Are you sure it was the 33rd floor?" he asked.

"I'm not positive. It was really late. Do you mind trying the 31st or 32nd floor?"

"No problem," he said.

It had become a challenge for him. He was going to continue searching. He brought out another stack of reservation slips and read off more names until he finally said, "Sue Piers. Palo Alto, California."

"That's it!" I said. "Thank you. Is there a phone number?"

"No. No phone number, but you could probably call information."

I thanked him heartily. He laughed and wished me luck as I walked toward the telephones, probably figuring I had had a one night stand that I wished I'd never had. But all directory assistance gave me was a couple of wrong numbers in Palo Alto and Menlo Park.

I left the hotel and drove back to Walnut Creek wondering what my next step should be. The Walnut Creek library was a few blocks from my apartment, so I got up on Saturday morning and decided to go over and do some more research in the hopes of tracking Sue down. Sure enough, Casto Travel, the agency she told me she worked for, and that suddenly re-registered for me, was listed in the Bay Area yellow pages.

*   *   *

When Monday rolled around I couldn't wait to call her. Two weeks had gone by, and I thought that if I didn't talk to her soon, any spark she'd felt for me might be gone.

I made the call.

"Hello. Casto Travel. May I help you?"

"Sue Piers please."

"One moment."

"Hi. This is Sue."

"Hi, Sue. This is Terry Healey. I don't know if you remember me, but I met you a couple weeks ago at Perry's Bar."

"Of course I remember. Can you hold for a second?"

A moment later she was back on the line. "How are you doing?"

"I'm great. And you?"

"Great. You know what? I'm late for a meeting. Can I get your number and call you back later today?"

"Sure." I gave her my number, sure that she was just making up an excuse so that she wouldn't have to talk to me.

'Oh, well,' I said to myself as I hung up. 'At least I tried.'

Around noon, about two hours later, my phone rang. It was Sue. We talked for about forty-five minutes and really hit it off, just as we had the first night we'd met.

I asked her if she would be interested in having a drink, and we decided to meet at Bix Restaurant in San Francisco that Friday at about six-thirty.

After a very long week, I arrived at the bar at six-thirty but saw no one resembling Sue. I bought myself a beer. A few minutes later I saw a woman walking toward me. She resembled Sue, but I didn't remember her hair being short or curly. Then she smiled, and I remembered that smile well. It was Sue. Thank God she had spotted me. She had permed her hair since I had last seen her, but she looked great.

We had a great evening together. That night, she never asked me what had happened to my face. I was sure I hadn't told her the first night in the city either. It seemed as if she really didn't care. Sue liked me for who I was. I was so interested in her that I forgot to tell her about myself.

*   *   *

Sue and I dated for about two years. After two years we bought a house together. I proposed to her two months later and we were married in September of 1994.

My life didn't really seem complete until I started dating Sue. I had started writing this book several months before meeting her, but she had brought so much joy and happiness to my life that I discarded the book, hoping some day I would get back to it. We worked hard and spent as much free time together as we could.

Marrying Sue changed everything. It closed the chapter in my life about my cancer and my personal struggles and insecurities. I suppose I will always be conscious of my defects, but I have learned to accept who I am.

I am now in a position to give back something to those struggling with cancer and disfigurement. I continue to volunteer at the Wellness Community and serve on their San Francisco Bay Area board of directors. I hope that somehow my words and experience can inspire others fighting for their lives and struggling with the mental, spiritual, emotional and physical challenges that cancer and disfigurement present to many of us.

After all, it is the internal and not the external fabric that makes up the human spirit. It is what lies beneath our skin that makes us unique. If each of us could focus on looking beyond the color of someone's skin or the appearance of someone's body or face, and instead focus on the person inside, our world would become a happier and more peaceful place.

Printed in the United States
732000001B